BACK PAIN
UNLOCKED

BACK PAIN UNLOCKED

ACHIEVE A PAIN-FREE FUNCTIONAL BACK USING THE BACK PAIN UNLOCKED System™

DR. LEX GONZALES, PT, DPT

BACK PAIN UNLOCKED:

ACHIEVE A PAIN-FREE FUNCTIONAL BACK USING THE BACK PAIN
UNLOCKED System™

The research and evidence-based information the author provided regarding the
subject covered should supplement rather than replace the advice of your physician
or physical/physiotherapist. Information contained within this book is not to be
construed as medical guidance. If you know or suspect you have a health problem,
consult your physician before embarking on any medical program, treatment, or
exercise regimen.

Design and cover art by Dr. Lex Gonzales, PT, DPT
Photography by Cecile+Lexi+Ani

Disclaimer: The author and publisher make no guarantees to the results you'll
achieve by reading this book. The information in this book is intended to provide
helpful and informative material on the subject addressed. It is not intended to serve
as a replacement for professional medical advice. Any use of the information in this
book is at the reader's discretion. The author and publisher specifically disclaim any
and all liability arising directly and indirectly from the use or application of any
information contained in this book. A healthcare professional should be consulted
regarding your specific situation.

Table of Contents

What good is being pain-free if you cannot function?
To what benefit is being able to function when it causes you pain?
I dedicate this book to those who want the best of both—
the ability to function without back pain.

DR. LEX GONZALES, PT, DPT

"All you need is the plan, the road map, and the courage to press on to your destination."

EARL NIGHTINGALE

Introduction

This Book Is For You

Do you suffer from chronic low back pain? Is it affecting your life in ways that are making you miserable? Do you need help to get rid of this problem once and for all? If so, **BACK PAIN UNLOCKED:** Achieve a Pain-Free Functional Back Using the Back Pain Unlocked System™ is the book for you.

You will find practical information on how to prevent and treat back pain in a clearly defined framework you can do at home. The *Back Pain Unlocked System™* is a coordinated and comprehensive framework that has helped many of my patients with their chronic low back pain problems, and now it can help YOU!

If you are looking to:

- Learn how to prevent and eliminate back pain without drugs, injections, or surgery.

- Know what exercises are good for you, why, and how.

- A guide to the most effective, safest, and quickest ways to help your back pain at home.

- A comprehensive, informative, and educational book.

- Evidence-based information from scientific studies.

- Reclaim your life from the grip of chronic low back pain.

Then this book is for you.

Skeptics read this: Treating back pain at home is not easy or quick. But it is possible.

- Have you tried different treatment modalities and seen different experts–doctors, therapists, chiropractors, acupuncturists, etc. and still haven't found a solution for your back pain?

- Have you tried drugs, injections, and even surgery but none of those worked for you?

- Have you tried several exercise programs but didn't understand the rhyme or reason for doing them?

- Are you willing to put in the time and effort to finally win your battle against chronic low back pain?

Then this book is for you, too.

This Book Is Not For You

In the vast majority of people experiencing chronic low back pain, symptoms can be attributed to nonspecific mechanical factors. However, in a much smaller percentage of people, the cause of back pain may be something more serious.

Conditions such as cancer, spinal compression or stress fractures, spinal infection, cauda equina syndromes, ankylosing spondylitis, or abdominal aortic aneurysm may sometimes present with symptoms that could be mistaken for low back pain.

If you are experiencing unrelenting constant pain that interferes with your sleep, and/or accompanies an unanticipated weight loss, these could be symptoms commonly referred to as red flags that require a thorough medical examination. If you suspect or have been diagnosed with these conditions, this book is not for you.

Why This Book is Different

Many people suffer from chronic low back pain and don't know what to do about it. They're often left feeling lost, confused, or frustrated when they can't figure out how to get relief.

It is not surprising that there are so many books written about chronic low back pain; however, most books focus on just one area - mostly exercises for your back - which may work well but doesn't offer readers the holistic framework they need.

Back Pain Unlocked begins with education and ends in implementation. *There is power in knowing why you do what you do.*

Parts 1 and 2 will provide you with a road map that will help you understand the complexity of pain. In Part 3, you will "walk the map" towards recovery.

Throughout these pages, I'm going to introduce you to the *Back Pain Unlocked System*™, a comprehensive framework I developed after working with adults suffering from varying degrees of chronic low back pain and dysfunction. When other methodologies and treatment modalities failed, I found that the *Back Pain Unlocked System*™ helped my patients achieve breakthroughs they had been badly looking for.

This book exists for one reason:

To provide you with a sensible solution to your back pain.

To do that, I've structured this book as follows:

First, I want to give you evidence-based information and scientific studies regarding the three most common medical interventions used to treat chronic low back pain today. Treatment interventions that are likely familiar to you, you may be currently using, or you are contemplating on availing soon.

I'll be asking self-assessment questions to help you make an informed decision on which treatment to take and help you know how to best proceed with your treatment intervention of choice.

After that, I'll make a case for how inherently strong your back is, and why the imaging studies containing those scary-sounding medical terminologies have nothing to do with the pain and dysfunction you are currently experiencing.

Next, I will untangle and simplify the complex neuroscience of pain. And don't worry, you do not need a doctorate-level degree to understand the otherwise complex study of pain. Before teaching it to my patients, I first practiced teaching it to my 5th-grade daughter to see if she would understand. She did. I am confident you will.

Finally, we'll spend a lot of time learning the *Back Pain Unlocked System*™. This is the system I developed after over twenty-four years of working with older adults suffering from varying degrees of chronic low back pain. I will show you how and why it worked so well for my patients.

The system you are about to discover allowed my patients to free themselves from the grip of pain and dysfunction. It is the same system that allowed my patients to win their lives back from their expressed misery. It is the same system that allowed them to live their best selves - achieving the quality of life they richly deserved!

The goal is for you to achieve a pain-free functional back.

Above all, I hope you learn not just the information but also the skills I'll be sharing with you in **Back Pain Unlocked**.

I sincerely believe that the more my patients know about their condition, the better able they are in helping themselves. I've seen the veracity of that belief in my clinical practice - the more I teach my patients about their health, the more empowered they are in taking care of themselves. The more they know, the healthier they become.

So, I consider it a great privilege to share with you what I have learned over the last twenty-four years of clinical practice. I hope it inspires you to know that there is an answer - that there is hope - that there is a sensible solution to your pain and dysfunction.

If you decide you'd like help to implement the *Back Pain Unlocked System*™, you can book a call to chat with my team by going to:

BPUsystem.com/call

You will master the knowledge and skills necessary while receiving the accountability to ensure your compliance and application of the *Back Pain Unlocked System*™ will help you achieve your own pain-free functional back.

We're here to help.

Your friend,

Dr. Lex Gonzales, PT, DPT

P.S. At the back of the book, I added a glossary of terms and their definitions to help you understand medical terminology that may be unfamiliar to you.

P.S.S. I also added a list of source materials composed of high-quality scientific research and evidence-based information if you want to dig deeper into the academic research and science I cite in this book.

*To protect patient privacy and confidentiality, names have been changed.

Part 1
THE CURRENT SOLUTION

Chapter 1

What Are Your Treatment Options?

"There are some remedies worse than the disease."

PUBLILIUS SYRUS

THE TIME HAS come for you to stop and think and look at yourself. If you are open to the notion that there should be a better way than being dependent on prescription pain medications, epidural spinal injections, or surgical knives and screws, then I urge you to pause from reading this book and look at yourself in the mirror.

Study yourself in the mirror. Look at your posture. Is your head protruding forward like a magnificent cobra about to strike its prey? Is one shoulder higher or lower than the other? What about your hips? Are they parallel and even? Is your upper back hunched over? Do your buttocks push out or sink in?

Now start moving. Study how you move. As you step back away from the mirror, were your steps fluid, or were you taking slow, uneven, painful steps? As you walk back toward the mirror, were your hips going up and down, or did you see a nice, even pattern of your hips or belly button floating toward the mirror? Go ahead, look now.

Your body, and how it moves in space, will tell you a story. Your body will be honest with you. With all the medications, injections, and possibly surgery you've had so far, is the body looking back at you in the mirror well?

Your body was made to move, not be numbed.

I have had the opportunity to work with patients in varying degrees of pain and dysfunction for over 24 years and have seen far too many who got lost in the medical rabbit's hole looking for answers to their back pain problems.

Indeed, there are several treatment options you can choose from to treat your back pain.

Study each one.

The success, or failure, of the treatment intervention you choose, will have long-term implications for your back in particular and for your overall health, in general.

WARNING:
Read and study the evidence
presented below before deciding
on a course of action.

PAIN MEDICATIONS

It must be confusing for you to have gone through different doctors only to be handed a prescription for a different pain medication each time; hoping that the medication they gave you will finally be the one to cure the pain.

Surely, pain medications, especially in the acute phase of low back pain (less than 3 months onset), are helpful in managing the pain. Using pain medications to manage pain in the acute phase will allow you to move and get back to your normal routine sooner.

However, it is time for you to look at the evidence on the long-term use of pain medications as the treatment of choice for treating chronic low back pain.

Time and time again, studies have shown the adverse effects of medication misuse and dependence on treating back pain.[1] As many choose to simply ingest a pill, they don't realize the adverse consequences to their mind and body until it is too late.

With continued use of opioid pain medications, (Fentanyl, Codeine, Lortab, Norco, Vicodin, Dilaudid, Demerol, Methadone, MS Contin, Oxycontin, Percocet, and a host of other generic and brand-name opioids) your body will adapt to these drugs and develop increasing tolerance to its effects.

Increasing drug tolerance means that you will need a higher dose of the drug to achieve the same level of response or relief your body achieved when you first started taking it. Your brain will send out signals it needs more opioids to feel good. The more you use the drug, the more your body builds a need for higher doses to feel any effect.

Pain is a message.

It is our brain and body's way of communicating to each other, telling each other, *"Hey, there's an actual or perceived threat to the body!"*

When you take a pain pill, you are ignoring the *reason* for the message. The medication will numb or dull away the message. As the effect of the medication wears off, the pain will persist, as long as the actual or perceived threat to your body remains.

Increased frequency of symptoms requires an increased frequency of pain medication use. Higher tolerance to the effect of the medication requires higher dosages.

That is how the cycle of pain results in medication dependency, or worse, addiction.

Why is this cycle perpetuated?

Because pain medications treat the symptom (the message) of low back pain, not the cause.

Why don't people just stop taking these opioid pain medications?

Because it is not easy to quit cold turkey.

Withdrawal from prolonged opioid pain medication use can induce restlessness, insomnia, diarrhea, vomiting, and increased sensitivity to pain. Through a variety of mechanisms, opioids cause adverse events in several organ systems in the body.[2-3]

According to the 2015 National Survey on Drug Use and Health (NSDUH), over one-third (37.8%) of the adult population in the US took prescription pain relievers.[3]

If these medications were effective in treating chronic low back pain, the United States wouldn't have the current crises and epidemic of opioid dependence and misuse.[4]

Consider these statistics from the U.S. Department of Health and Human Services:[5]

THE OPIOID EPIDEMIC BY THE NUMBERS

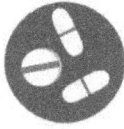

130+
People died every day from
opioid-related drug overdoses[3]
(estimated)

11.4 m
People misused
prescription opioids[1]

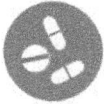

47,600
People died from
overdosing on opioids[2]

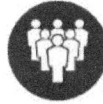

2.1 million
People had an opioid use
disorder[1]

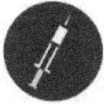

81,000
People used heroin
for the first time[1]

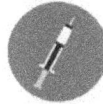

886,000
People used heroin[1]

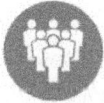

2 million
People misused prescription
opioids for the first time[1]

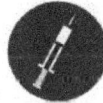

15,482
Deaths attributed to
overdosing on heroin[2]

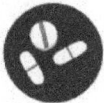

28,466
Deaths attributed to
overdosing on synthetic
opioids other than methadone[2]

SOURCES
1. 2017 National Survey on Drug Use and Health, Mortality in the United States, 2016
2. NCHS Data Brief No. 293, December 2017
3. NCHS, National Vital Statistics System. Estimates for 2017 and 2018 are based on provisional data.

Updated January 2019. For more information, visit: http://www.hhs.gov/opioids/   HHS.GOV/OPIOIDS

After decades of increasing dependence and abuse of opioid pain medications, in 2016 the US Centers for Disease Control and Prevention (CDC) released the *"Guideline for Prescribing Opioids for Chronic Pain"*.

The guideline is intended to improve communication between clinicians and patients about the risks and benefits of opioid therapy, and to chart a safer, more effective course on the use of opioids for treating chronic pain.

Here is the number one recommendation listed on the CDC guideline:

#1. Nonpharmacologic therapy and non-opioid pharmacological therapy are preferred for chronic pain.[6]

The guideline included the following statement: "*In the past decade, while the death rates for the top leading causes of death such as heart disease and cancer have decreased substantially, the death rate associated with opioid pain medication has increased markedly.*"

During the earlier, or acute stages of back pain, pain medications can be a temporary approach to help reduce the pain and calm the muscle spasms frequently accompanying back pain. Once your back pain eases, medication use should be tapered down and ultimately stopped.

Medication use is not meant to "ward off" the pain so that the pain "will not come back".

Before starting with opioid pain medications to treat your chronic low back pain, ask your doctor, "*What is the plan to taper off these medications?*"

EPIDURAL STEROID INJECTIONS

Years ago, I received a referral for a 72-year-old patient with a diagnosis of lumbar strain. The patient reported that she hurt her back after bending down to pick up her cat. Prior to my evaluation, my initial hunch, based on the referral, was that she may have just "pulled" her back muscles when she bent down to the floor to pick up her cat.

After my evaluation, it was evident that my patient had more than just "pulled" her back muscles. I sent her back to her primary doctor with a request for an X-ray. I suspected she had a vertebral fracture, not a lumbar strain, as the diagnosis on her referral says.

Five days later, I received word that she was admitted to the hospital; recovering from surgery for her T12 and L1 vertebra compression fracture.

What made me suspect that my patient had a fracture in her spine prior to her getting an X-ray?

When I interviewed my patient during my initial evaluation, she mentioned she has had multiple epidural steroid injections over the years to treat her chronic low back pain.

I knew of the adverse effect of prolonged steroid use.

Glucocorticoids, the steroid used in epidural injections to reduce pain and inflammation, could make bones fragile, a condition known as *glucocorticoid-induced osteoporosis* or GIO. GIO is a serious consequence of glucocorticoid therapy leading to osteoporotic fractures in 30-50% of patients.[7]

In 2012, Shlomo Mandel, an internal medicine specialist at Henry Ford Health System, led a team that investigated the effects of epidural steroid injections among women over the age of sixty-five.

What they found was that for *each* epidural steroid injection administered, the risk of vertebral compression fracture increased by 21%.[8]

In 2014, the U.S. Food and Drug Administration (FDA), released a Drug Safety Communication, with the following announcement, "*The U.S. Food and Drug Administration (FDA) is warning that injection of corticosteroids into the* epidural space *of the spine may result in rare but serious adverse events, including loss of vision, stroke, paralysis, and death.*"[9]

In 2015, the Agency for Healthcare Research and Quality (AHRQ) reviewed the medical literature and made the following conclusion:

"*Epidural corticosteroid injections for* radiculopathy *were associated with immediate improvements in pain and might be associated with immediate improvements in function, but benefits were small and not sustained, and there was no effect on long-term risk of surgery.*

Evidence did not suggest that effectiveness varies based on injection technique, corticosteroid, dose, or comparator. Limited evidence suggested that epidural corticosteroid injections are not effective for spinal stenosis or non-radicular back pain and that facet joint corticosteroid injections are not effective for presumed facet joint pain. There was insufficient evidence to evaluate effectiveness of sacroiliac joint corticosteroid injections." [10]

With its perceived benefit in question and the risks to long-term health high, I recommend that you have an ample discussion with your doctor prior to getting a shot on your back.

I encourage you to ask, *"Are the risks worth the benefits?"*

SPINAL SURGERY

1. Are you losing sensation in your buttocks or your limbs?
2. Have you noticed your limbs getting weaker?
3. Are you having difficulty coordinating the movement of your feet?
4. Are you having difficulty controlling your ability to urinate or move your bowel?

Unless you have worsening neurologic symptoms listed above, back pain, in and of itself, should not be an indication for surgery.

In the summer of 2015, Steve Kerr, an accomplished professional basketball player, and later, head coach in the National Basketball Association (NBA), underwent spinal surgery to repair a herniated disc on his back.

Soon after the surgery, Kerr experienced debilitating headaches, nausea, and a host of other new problems. ESPN's Ramona Shelbourne reported, *"For months, he was a shell of himself, battling intense pressure headaches and searing pain behind his eyes. He felt sick, weak, tired, and dizzy."* [11]

After going back and forth among different medical specialists, Kerr found out the reason behind the new set of symptoms he was experiencing: the membrane covering his spinal cord was punctured during his spinal surgery, causing his cerebrospinal fluid (CSF) to leak.

That fall, Kerr underwent a second spinal surgery to repair the problem caused by the first spinal surgery. The second surgery did not successfully correct the problem.

Once you open up your back for surgery, there is no undoing what has been done. Whether good or bad.

So many patients decide on having surgery without ample discussion with their doctors on the data and evidence regarding the efficacy of surgery in treating chronic low back pain.

In the Popular Lectures and Addresses series, mathematician and physicist William Thomson explained this process bluntly, *"When you can measure what you are speaking about, and express it in numbers, you know something about it; but when you cannot measure it, your knowledge is of a meager and unsatisfactory kind."*[12]

Simply said, if you cannot tie a specific piece of data to the conclusion you are drawing, then you are simply guessing.

The data from the Agency for Healthcare Research and Quality (AHRQ) revealed that, in 2011, there were 490,000 laminectomies performed in the United States, and between 2001 and 2011 there was a 70 percent increase in spinal fusion surgeries, from 287,000 to 488,300.[13]

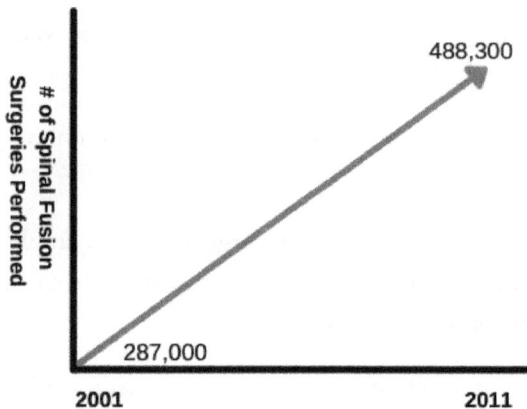

Figure 1. Increase in Spinal Fusion Surgeries Performed in 10 years

This increased rate of spinal surgeries, unfortunately, did not correspond to an increase in successful outcomes. On the contrary, a conservative estimate of 20 percent, with other estimates as high as 40 percent, of these surgeries have failed to treat the pain.[14]

Failure of surgery to resolve the pain is such a common consequence that a term has been coined to describe the condition: *Failed Back Surgery Syndrome* (FBSS).

The International Association for the Study of Pain defines failed back surgery syndrome (FBSS) as:

Lumbar spinal pain of unknown origin either persisting despite surgical intervention or appearing after surgical intervention for spinal pain originally in the same topographical location.[15]

In other words, the surgery designed to relieve the pain has not resolved the pain, or the pain has recurred just as it was before surgery.

According to the American Journal of Medicine, in the United States alone, about 80,000 spine surgeries fail *annually*.[16]

Two years after his failed back surgery and after undergoing intensive physi-cal/physiotherapy, Washington Post reported Kerr offering his advice to those who have back problems, *"I can tell you if you're listening out there, stay away from back surgery. I can say that from the bottom of my heart. Rehab, rehab, rehab. Don't let anyone get in there."* [17]

At the conference of the American Academy of Orthopedic Surgeons in 2010, a hundred surgeons were asked whether they themselves will undergo lumbar spinal fusion surgery for nonspecific low back pain.

Ninety-nine out of the one hundred surgeons answered, *"Absolutely not."* [18]

There are imperative reasons why surgery is indicated. Pain, by and of itself, is not. Make an educated and informed decision by having an ample discus-sion with your doctor.

If your doctor recommends surgery to treat your back pain, ask, *"If you have the same condition as my back, would you undergo the same surgical procedure you are recommending?*

YOUR NEW OPPORTUNITY

Modern society has lulled us into using these "quick fixes" - a pill, an injec-tion, even surgery. Unfortunately, many people are not aware of the adverse consequences as described by the multiple studies you've just read.

In my experience, patients refrain from moving their bodies not because they don't want to, but because they do not know how to. They are mostly afraid that moving a painful part of their body, particularly their back, will only cause more pain. Understandably, it is often hard to stay active if you are in pain. Our natural inclination will be to stay still, or to stay in bed, not moving a limb, for fear that movement will aggravate the pain.

We need to correct that notion here and now:

> *"Not moving, in order for your low back pain to get better, is a myth."*

Multiple research studies have shown that not moving enough can worsen your back pain, not resolve the problem. A systematic review of studies for the management of back pain has recommendations for more, rather than less activity in recovery.[19-20]

Long periods of inactivity, or lack of movement, will adversely affect your recovery from back pain.[21-22]

As you restrict the movement of your trunk, you further reduce the strength of your core and increase your lumbar instability, resulting in more back pain, not less.[23]

Weakening of your abdominal muscles can also tilt your pelvis posteriorly and can result in even more back pain.[24,25]

Restricting your movement, over time, will also affect the flexibility of your muscles and cause more back pain.[26]

The more you stay still, or sit around, or stay in bed, the worse your back pain gets. What Sir Isaac Newton said about the first law of physics is just as true with the human body, *"A body in motion stays in motion. A body at rest stays at rest."*

In the *Back Pain Unlocked System*™, I will teach you the framework I developed to guide my patients through the different areas needed to improve their pain and function.

An exercise handout is not the universal remedy for back pain.

The *Back Pain Unlocked System*™ recognizes that back exercises are an important part of your recovery. But it is just one part.

The *Back Pain Unlocked System*™ further recognizes that pain is a multidimensional experience. Yes, there is the physical aspect of your experience that we need to address with postural and movement retraining and exercises. But exercises alone will not suffice. We must recognize that there are psychological, behavioral, and emotional aspects to the pain experience. And these factors are also affected and informed by your social function and experiences.[27-28]

If you have already tried several back exercise programs and failed, it is not your fault. Like a three-legged stool, you need the other two components of the *Back Pain Unlocked System*™ to succeed. Take off one leg of the stool and you'll come crashing down from the weight of your chronic low back pain.

In the pages of this book, I will outline as best as I can the different components at play in your recovery using the *Back Pain Unlocked System*™. It's possible that a simple, short book could be what you have been looking for to finally unlock the ideas and strategies you've been missing all along in your search for a long-term solution to your chronic low back pain and dysfunction.

If you want to radically transform your pain and dysfunction into fitness and function, learn the *Back Pain Unlocked System*™.

Chapter 2

The Mistake Almost
Everybody Makes

"Admitting we're wrong is courage, not weakness."

Roy T. Bennett

CONSIDERING HOW COMMON low back pain is, and with so many books written about it *(not to mention the abundance of free information available online)*, one would think that it would be easy to know the difference between *acute* and *chronic* low back pain.

After listening to many of my patients, however, I came to recognize and appreciate the fact that knowing and understanding the difference between the two is not that easy.

The same interaction with many of my patients also brought home to me the distressing reality that many healthcare providers, including doctors, chiropractors, physical therapists, and other clinicians specializing in bodywork, continue to treat both acute and chronic back pain conditions the same way.

There is either a lack of recognition of the differences between the two or a lack of understanding that each one needs to be treated differently.

There are different definitions in the literature, but the commonly accepted definitions for the duration of low back pain symptoms are:[1]

1. Acute - less than 1 month.

2. Subacute - between 2 and 3 months.

3. Chronic - over 3 months since initial onset of pain and symptoms.

As you can see, the variability in how long you've had your low back pain, whether it is *acute*, *subacute*, or *chronic*, will influence a lot of the decisions on how to treat your back pain.

This is when it can get confusing for a lot of patients.

Imagine each distinct step you'll have to take on your journey to recovery:

1. The initial episode of your low back pain.

2. Call and schedule an appointment with your primary doctor.

3. Meet with your primary doctor.

4. Your primary doctor requests an imaging study, e.g., X-ray, MRI, etc.

5. Call and schedule your X-ray or MRI appointment.

6. Your primary doctor receives your X-ray or MRI result.

7. Depending on your medical imaging result, your primary doctor either prescribes you pain medications, refers you to physical therapy, and/or refers you to an orthopedic or pain doctor.

8. Call and schedule an appointment with the orthopedic or pain doctor or physical therapist.

9. Meet with your orthopedic or pain doctor.

10. Meet with your physical therapist.

11. FINALLY, receive treatment for your low back pain.

From the time you initially experienced low back pain symptoms to the time it takes one healthcare professional to refer you to another, you may already have gone through the whole continuum of the back pain duration.

We're supposed to treat back pain differently in each of the different stages but rarely is a patient in the United States treated by just one healthcare professional over the course of their care.

No wonder why so many people are frustrated with the course of their back pain treatment!

Acute vs Chronic Low Back Pain

While there are many potential causes of acute low back pain, most of them have no serious underlying causes. In the vast majority of patients with acute low back pain, we can attribute symptoms to *nonspecific mechanical factors.*

Nonspecific mechanical factors are back pain that stems from the spine, intervertebral disks, or surrounding soft tissues. This includes muscle strain, disk herniation, lumbar spondylosis, and acute or repetitive traumatic injury.

These mechanical factors can result from:

- Injury from exercise, heavy lifting, or a sudden and awkward movement.
- Muscle spasms.
- Trauma from a fall or vehicle accident.
- Osteoporosis or minor compression fractures.
- Arthritis causing the hollow opening around the spinal cord or nerves to narrow.
- Bulging or herniated discs.
- Repetitive trauma and overuse injuries.

Acute low back pain develops suddenly, often because of an identifiable injury, and will either heal spontaneously or respond to the usual medical and physical therapy treatments you are familiar with.

In most cases, acute low back pain caused by nonspecific mechanical factors will not become chronic.

In contrast, most chronic low back pain, though may initially be caused by structural or mechanical factors, does not develop from physical or structural causes but is rather caused by *neuroplastic pain.*[2]

To better understand neuroplasticity, let us break it down into its root words:

neuro = brain

plasticity = the ability of neural networks to change through growth and reorganization.

In other words, neuroplasticity refers to your brain's ability to change and adapt as a result of your experience.

With neuroplastic pain, you still feel pain even when there is no damage to the body or even after the initial injury has already healed.

Pain caused by neuroplasticity occurs when the brain interprets messages from the body as danger signals. (*Learn more about the "living pain alarm system" in Chapter 8.*)

Occasionally, patients may suffer from chronic low back pain for structural or physical reasons. These conditions, however, may sometimes present with symptoms that look like low back pain, but maybe much more serious and require a thorough medical examination.

Serious medical conditions that may be mistaken for back pain include:

- Cancer
- Spinal compression or stress fractures
- Spinal infection

- Cauda equina syndrome

- Ankylosing spondylitis

- Abdominal aortic aneurysm

If you are experiencing unrelenting or constant back pain that interferes with your sleep, and/or accompanies an unanticipated weight loss, these could be symptoms commonly referred to as red flags. See your doctor and ask for a thorough medical evaluation.

Following a thorough medical evaluation, if these red flag conditions have been eliminated, it is highly likely that your back pain is caused by neuro-plastic pain.

Do Not Repeat This Mistake

As you can see, acute and chronic low back pain have very different causes and should therefore be treated differently.

Remember, acute low back pain from structural causes heals fairly quickly. Follow a well-coordinated back exercise program to advance and maintain your recovery (see the ASM Roadmap of the Back Pain Unlocked System™ in Chapter 9).

While acute low back is mostly mechanical or structural, most chronic low back pain is neuroplastic in nature.

When you have had persistent or recurring low back pain for over 3 months and all red flag conditions have been eliminated, addressing not just the physical but also the psychological and social factors impacting your pain experience is the most sensible and effective way to treat your back pain.

With neuroplastic pain causing most chronic low back pain, it is very important to use a comprehensive back program to address the different factors contributing to your experience of pain.

The latest evidence and studies on the neuroscience of pain have proven the efficacy of brain training, graded motor imagery, meditation, visualization, somatic tracking, and other cognitive-behavioral techniques in treating chronic pain conditions, including chronic low back pain.[3]

Back Pain Unlocked System™ addresses the different factors associated with your pain by using the biopsychosocial model of treatment.

Chapter 3

Who This Book (And System) Is For

"Don't wait for an opportunity. Create it."

GEORGE BERNARD SHAW

The system you are about to learn is the result of fourteen words I heard over eighteen years ago. To this day, I can still feel how I felt then when I first heard those words.

I just started working as a licensed physical therapist here in the United States. I was young, inexperienced, nervous - yet confident. I was confident that five years of study and clinical assignments had prepared me exactly for such a time as this. I have read thousands of pages of textbooks and researched countless studies on how to treat back pain.

I *know* how to treat back pain.

I carefully deliberated each movement and exercise I prescribed to Martha*, a 68-year-old lady whose springy gait and demeanor were replaced by slow, painful steps. Her body, frozen in a forward-bent position, slumped on her walker.

I worked with Martha for over five weeks, treating her back pain and help-ing her to regain her function and independence. One balmy morning, she came in early for her appointment and told me the words that sucked the wind off that spring morning.

She uttered fourteen words that haunted me and how I treat my patients ever since. She said, *"Lex, my back pain has not improved… I scheduled myself for a back surgery."*

I felt Martha's pain and anguish. I felt my failure and disappointment.

Why didn't Martha's back pain get better?

I followed all the exercise protocols and techniques preached by the text-books I studied in school. Why did it not work?

Those questions haunted me. I wanted to know how to help my next patient. I wanted to help my next Martha. I want my patients to get better. I don't want my patients to give up or resign themselves to a life of pain and quiet desperation.

I spent the next decade of my physical therapy practice looking for answers. It culminated in my going back to school to pursue a doctorate degree in physical therapy.

I've worked with hundreds of patients suffering from back pain since Martha. I've since used best practices and clinical guidelines to achieve the best possible outcomes for my patients.

I've seen what works.

I've also seen what doesn't work.

The ones that worked and helped my patients the most, I refined even more. I sharpened the techniques and studied some more.

I listened to what my patients have told me.

And here I'll share with you the first important lesson:

No matter what exercise protocol or technique is used, not all chronic low back pain can be remedied by exercise alone.

I made the mistake of forgetting the most important member of the recovery team - the patient. I taught my patients the exercise protocols and techniques, and just like a well-meaning and aggressive coach, pushed them to perform to the best of what I know they are capable of. But I forgot to listen to what they really were thinking about the pain they're experiencing.

From the outside looking in, they may follow the exercises I prescribed but if they continue to subscribe to negative beliefs, catastrophizing their pain, and avoiding normal movements and activities because of fear, they will continue to experience pain.

In the past two decades, clinical researchers have unraveled the significant role certain specific sets of negative beliefs play in an individual's pain experience.[1]

Indeed, there is a strong connection between how you think and how you feel. It is usually not what happens to you that makes you feel anxious or tense, but what you tell yourself about your experience.

When you are worried or are in a stressful situation, you might have lots of thoughts about the situation that often make you think differently than you would normally do.

These distorted belief systems often involve catastrophic thoughts, overestimating the degree of emotional distress and discomfort, or overly focusing on the negative aspects of pain caused by the injury.[2]

Since implementing the *Back Pain Unlocked System*™, there have been three specific improvements I see my patients achieve:

One, by recognizing their own belief systems, they are better equipped to anticipate their reactions to the stresses that would otherwise aggravate their pain. By embedding prompts for brain training, writing, meditation, or guided visualization into the *Back Pain Unlocked System*™, you can overcome and change your maladaptive beliefs about pain.

Two, by understanding the inherent structural strength of their back, they start to trust themselves and their body's capacity to heal. An integral part of the *Back Pain Unlocked System*™ is the education you get. Gone are the days of exercising for the sake of exercising. That old road leads nowhere. You must know why you do what you do.

Three, by baking in accountability cues to action, they are more likely to stay the course and see themselves through their goals. Not knowing other people undergoing the same problem as you do can be isolating. Yes, you have your circle of friends and family that can support you, but do you have somebody in that circle making sure that you follow your exercise program? Somebody who holds you accountable for what you said you will do today. Or tomorrow. Every day?

One of the most powerful things you can do today is to be purposeful in evaluating your beliefs about your own pain experience. Drill down to what makes you scared to do what you used to do with ease. Are you afraid your back will not hold up?

Are you being intentional in surrounding yourself with people who can help you recover from your injury and pain, or are they instead adding to your stress and worry, aggravating your pain experience even more?

I am not saying you should forgo the people not helping you. What I am saying is to identify those who can help you and make you accountable for the results you are trying to achieve.

You will find, once you finish this book and put it into action, that by gaining clarity on your belief system, understanding the inherent strength and capacity of your back, and sticking it through with your program, you'll break free from your pain and enjoy the quality of life you richly deserve.

It is my sincere hope that by teaching you the *Back Pain Unlocked System*™, you will find an alternative to the medical rabbit hole of the "quick pain fixes" of pain medications, spinal injections, and surgery.

It is my sincere hope that by reading this short book, you will see a clear path toward a sensible solution to your chronic low back pain.

As you will see though, the *Back Pain Unlocked System*™ is not for everyone. If you are looking for a quick fix, the *Back Pain Unlocked System*™ is not for you.

I will teach you techniques to unlearn faulty postural habits and relearn new movement patterns. It requires focus and discipline - an investment of both time and energy. It is for people who have tried or are tired of depending on pain medications, injections, or surgery. It is for people looking for a sensible movement program to reclaim their life from chronic low back pain. It is for people willing to invest in themselves.

KEY CHAPTER TAKEAWAYS

- Exercise alone, though an integral part of your recovery, is not the cure-all for chronic low back pain. You need to evaluate your own belief systems toward pain. Delve into what makes you afraid to move. Ask, "*Other than the physical component, what other factors contribute to or aggravate my pain experience?*"

- Having a clear and foundational understanding of the inherent strength of your back can help you minimize your fear of movement. Not limiting your physical and social activities will help hasten your recovery.

- Humans are social beings. Having another person holding you accountable for the results you want to achieve makes it more likely for you to achieve those results.

Master the *Back Pain Unlocked System*™

Before we proceed with the rest of the book, let's first check-in with where you're at right now on your journey to a pain-free functional back.

Below, rate yourself on a scale from 1 - 10 on how accurate the statements are—1 means "not accurate at all," and 10 means "most accurate."

Once you've rated yourself for each statement, total up your scores and then use the Answer Key to determine your next steps.

Self-Assessment Statement	Self-Rating
I have an exercise program/protocol that works for me.	
I advocate for my own back pain treatment.	
I clearly understand the inherent anatomical/structural strength of my back.	
I clearly understand my own beliefs, feelings, and attitude towards my back pain experience.	
I can anticipate my response to stress and mitigate its effect on my back pain experience.	
I trust that my back is strong and capable of supporting my daily physical activities.	
I have people who hold me accountable to follow through with my back program.	
I have people who prompt me in case I forget to do my back exercises.	
I do not limit my physical or social activities because of back pain.	
I am not dependent on or looking for pain medications, injections, or surgery as the long-term solution to my chronic low back pain.	

What Your Score Really Means

Score: 0-55

The bad news is that you are missing foundational elements to help you achieve a long-term solution to your chronic low back pain. You probably already know this as you have been actively looking for solutions but haven't gotten a straight answer from your doctor, therapist, chiropractor, etc.

However, the good news is that all of that can be easily solved, and even better, it means that by reading this book, you get to support your foundational knowledge with evidence-based information from quality research and studies.

Read this book with an open mind.

Consider how implementing **Back Pain Unlocked** from the ground up could radically improve your chronic low back pain for the better. It won't take much for you to experience a night and day improvement.

Score 56-75

If your score landed you here, it means that you have a good foundational solution to your chronic low back pain but are missing some key components to support a long-term solution.

You likely either have a clear understanding of the structural strength of your back but do not have an effective back exercise program or you do have a back exercise program working for you but do not have a good accountability system to ensure you follow through with the program.

As you will learn from this book, putting these different components together will significantly increase your chances of achieving a pain-free functional back.

Score 76+

You have a very good understanding of the inherent strength of your back, you have an effective back exercise program that works for you, and you have put in place a working accountability system.

Use what you will learn from this book to organize your back program into a comprehensive system and use the framework I developed to supercharge your program.

If your goal is to have a long-term solution to your chronic low back pain and achieve a pain-free functional back, then all you need to do is implement the system as shown in this book, and you'll be well on your way.

Chapter 4

Overcoming Your Biggest Hurdles

"Strength does not come from what you can do.
It comes from overcoming the things you once thought you couldn't."

Rikki Rogers

In over twenty-four years of working with adults suffering from varying degrees of chronic low back pain and dysfunction, I've learned a few things. Things one cannot learn from textbooks but only from being in the trenches, working and listening to patients and sharpening one's tools through the years.

I want to share with you the biggest hurdles you will face in your own journey to recovery for two reasons:

1. So you can learn from the lessons other people learned and apply those lessons to help you succeed in your own recovery.

2. To show you why the *Back Pain Unlocked System™* worked so well in helping them achieve a pain-free functional back.

I think you will find a tremendous amount of value in seeing the hurdles ahead of time and getting yourself ready for what you will face in your own journey from pain and dysfunction to personal power and freedom.

Let's talk about these hurdles:

Hurdle #1. Mind Matters

I once asked my patient, "Did you know that 80% of the people in the world experience back pain at some point in their life?[1]

Most people you know have either experienced back pain before, are currently suffering from it, or will have back pain in the future.

Just like the common cold, back pain is not a unique but a common experience of being human.[2]

My patient objected to what I said and added, "*I don't know about that. My back pain is different from those experienced by my friends and family. Mine is the worst.*"

I listened to my patient attentively, acknowledging that back pain is a sensation that most people have felt at some point in their lives. Many people know that. But what many people may not know and understand is just how pain works and why it is so hard to manage.

Whether it's from an injury, illness, or chronic condition, pain can make life difficult to live and work. It can be tough for many of us to understand the experience of living with chronic low back pain because most of the time we only think of the physical aspect of the pain when we think of back pain.

What you may not realize is that your thoughts, emotions, or behaviors contribute to your experience of pain. If you interpret pain as a threat and start to think about it all the time, you will be hypervigilant or over-monitoring of your bodily sensations. It will cascade down to excessive worry and even an inability to shift your attention away from pain-related thoughts.

For example, if you have back pain and then start to worry about being in pain or that the pain will never go away, it can lead to feeling afraid of doing things. Excessive worry, negative self-statements, and feelings of helplessness will make you feel like not moving much at all.

This is called catastrophizing and fear-avoidance behavior. You may develop negative expectations based on your previous memories of pain. You might feel helpless; unable to cope effectively with pain.[3-5]

Interestingly, pain catastrophizing has been found to intensify the experience of pain and depression. Higher pain catastrophizing is associated with higher self-reported pain and disability and may lead to delayed recovery in patients with low back pain.[6-7]

If you currently are experiencing chronic low back pain, recognize how your belief systems are informing your behavior. Are you keeping yourself from doing the usual activities you used to do before with ease?

If you hope to achieve a pain-free functional back, acknowledge that pain is not just a physical experience. Pain is a multidimensional experience. Know not just where you're feeling the pain or how bad your pain is, but recognize *what you think* about the pain, *how you feel* about the pain, and *how you react* to the pain.

Once you are clear with the inventory of your thoughts and emotions regarding your pain experience, utilize the tools baked-in in the *Back Pain Unlocked System*™. This is where you will discover the power of brain training, guided meditation, graded motor imagery, and even writing to turn down your hypersensitivity to pain.

Your brain and nervous system, through its property of plasticity, can be reprogrammed to perceive and process pain in a healthier manner.

Later in this book, I will show you the cognitive and behavioral components of the *Back Pain Unlocked System*™ - components integrated into the **Back Pain Unlocked** program.

For now, take a moment to check in with yourself.

Master the *Back Pain Unlocked System*™

Before we proceed with the rest of the book, let's first take an inventory of what you currently think, believe, or feel about your experience with pain.

Below, rate yourself on a scale from 1 - 10 on how accurate the statements are—1 means "not accurate at all," and 10 means "most accurate."

Once you've rated yourself for each statement, total up your scores and then use the Answer Key to determine your next steps.

Self-Assessment Statement	Self-Rating
I don't have feelings of helplessness, worry, or anxiety when I experience low back pain.	
I can look after myself and my daily needs without causing extra pain.	
Pain does not prevent me from walking any distance.	
My work does not aggravate my pain.	
Physical activities do not make my pain worse.	
My social life does not cause me extra pain.	

Score 0-25

Many factors, including your thoughts, beliefs, emotions, attitude, etc., inform your experience of pain. Because of the extended duration of your experience with pain, your brain became overprotective of your body. It interprets normal activities you used to do with ease as a threat, sending pain signals to prevent you from moving or taking part in physical activities.

Read the chapter on pain neuroscience and use the cognitive-behavioral tools I outlined in Part 3. This powerful information will help you reframe your pain experience and dial down the hypersensitivity of your nervous system's alarm system.

Score 26-45

Whether or not you were aware of it, you have developed some cognitive-behavioral tools to help mitigate the effects of pain in your daily life. For the most part, you have learned to not let pain dictate your ability to function. You just need to organize the tools in your cognitive-behavioral toolbox, so you'll know exactly which ones to pull out in the event low back pain threatens your ability to participate in physical activities.

Be clear with your ideas, beliefs, feelings, and attitude toward pain and your battle with chronic low back pain is already halfway won.

Score 46+

Congratulations, you have learned to perceive and process pain in a healthy manner! Study and use the other two legs of *The Back Pain Unlocked System*™. Having all three legs of a comprehensive back program supporting your recovery will give you a stable foundation and help you attain a long-term solution to your back pain.

Hurdle #2. Lack of Clarity

It is hard to hit a target with your eyes closed.

It might surprise you, but many people do not actually have a clear understanding of their back program, nor do they know the significance of the exercises they are doing relative to the goals they are trying to achieve.

Exercising for the sake of exercising is not a good treatment plan. It is like throwing spaghetti on the wall, hoping something will stick.

That is how people get disappointed with their back exercise programs. They don't know why they are doing what they are doing, nor do they have an idea of which point they are at in their journey to recovery.

Before starting a back exercise program, begin with the end in mind. Ask, *"What are you hoping to accomplish with the program you are following?*

Which exercise will get you the result you need at your particular stage of recovery?

Are you moving toward the direction you're wanting to go or are you doing unnecessary exercises and activities that are not geared toward your immediate need?"

Without a roadmap, how else are you going to know if you're going in the direction you want? Or how will you measure your incremental progress toward your goal?

Remember, **you are the most important member of the recovery team**. You *must* have a clear understanding of your back exercise program.

Also, in your zeal to do each exercise correctly, do not get lost in the details. Yes, accurate and safe execution of your exercises is important, but do not miss the forest for the trees. Know where you are in your journey of recovery and know how to get to your goal of achieving a pain-free functional back. Use a roadmap.

Later, I'll show you a roadmap you can follow and gain clarity on what you're trying to achieve.

For now, it's worth taking a moment to see where you are in your journey of recovery. Go ahead and take the assessment below.

Master the *Back Pain Unlocked System*™

Before we proceed with the rest of the book, let's first check how clear you are with the back program you are currently using.

Below, rate yourself on a scale from 1 - 10 on how accurate the statements are—1 means "not accurate at all," and 10 means "most accurate."

Once you've rated yourself for each statement, total up your scores and then use the Answer Key to determine your next steps.

Self-Assessment Statement	Self-Rating
I clearly understand what my current back program is trying to accomplish.	
I understand the reason why I am doing the exercises I am currently doing.	
I know which stage I am in my journey of recovery and the exercises I am doing are appropriate for my current stage.	
I have a clear mental picture of where I am and the direction I am going with my back program.	
With my current back program, I am able to measure my progress toward my goals.	
The exercises I am doing now reflect the level of mastery I have of the exercises from my previous stages of recovery.	

Score 0-35

It is not your fault if you do not have a clear understanding of what a back program should be and how it is supposed to help you. Our current healthcare environment is fragmented. Often, you have different doctors and other healthcare practitioners taking care of the different parts or systems of your body. Sadly, they don't always talk to each other.

Even more reason you should be the leading advocate for your own health care. Remember, you are the most important member of the recovery team.

In the area of chronic low back pain management, have a clear understanding of your back program. Use a roadmap to give yourself a "view" of where you are currently standing relative to where you want to go.

Use Chapter 8 to gain clarity on what you need to do to get to where you want to be.

Score 36-44

You know where you are in your journey to recovery. You just needed a hand to lead you where you wanted to go - freedom from pain and dysfunction.

Ask your physical therapist to organize your back exercise program in a manner that reflects your current needs, and that leads you to your goal of independence. Insist on having a "clear view of the road map".

Score 45+

It's time for you to systematize your back care program. You already know where you are and where you wanted to go in your exercise program. Use prompts and accountability partners to help you stick with your program.

Many people know where they are in their journey to recovery and what they need to do to get to where they want to be - a life free from pain and dysfunction. But knowing is not doing.

The social component of the Back Pain Unlocked System™ will give you the tools to assist with consistency and compliance, also one of the hurdles a lot of people face in their journey to recovery.

Hurdle #3. Mastering Movement

Are you familiar with *lumbopelvic motor control* and coordination exercises? What about *transversus abdominis* and *lumbar multifidus* activation and strengthening? Or dynamic lumbar stabilization exercises?

If you are not familiar with some of those terms, you are not alone. That is why I developed the *Back Pain Unlocked System*™ and wrote the **Back Pain Unlocked** book. Without the right information and guidance, people with chronic low back pain get victimized twice – first, by the dysfunction caused by their chronic low back pain and second, by the unintended consequence of "quick fix" solutions.

In their haste to treat their chronic low back pain, many people get started in the medical rabbit chase of opioid pain medications, epidural steroid injections, and ultimately, spinal surgery. Often, people get lost in the maze of confusing information.

Stop chasing the rabbit and take control of your back pain. The time has come for you to reclaim your personal power. The time has come for you to move your body the way it was made to. If you are serious about your goal to achieve a pain-free functional back, invest yourself in mastering correct movement patterns. You will learn skills that will benefit you for the rest of your life.

- Learn how to move your pelvis to position your spine in its optimal pain-free neutral position.

- Learn how to activate your core muscles to form a brace and support your spine.

- Learn how to coordinate the activation of your spinal muscles to stand the rigors required by your daily tasks and activities.

Here's why:

Taking part in a back program for an hour or two every day will not reverse the other twenty-two to twenty-three hours of faulty posture and movement patterns. Again, you are the most important member of the recovery team. What you do in your time away from your back program has more impact than what you achieve in that hour or two of treatment.

The first step is to master postural and movement patterns. Luckily, this book will show you how and you'll see how simple it can really be.

For now, see where you are in your knowledge and application of correct postural and movement patterns by doing the assessment below.

Master the *Back Pain Unlocked System*™

Before we proceed with the rest of the book, let's first take account of your knowledge and skill in mastering correct movement patterns that support and protect your back.

Below, rate yourself on a scale from 1 - 10 on how accurate the statements are—1 means "not accurate at all," and 10 means "most accurate."

Once you've rated yourself for each statement, total up your scores and then use the Answer Key to determine your next steps.

Self-Assessment Statement	Self-Rating
I know how to position my spine in its pain-free neutral position.	
I know how to activate my core muscles to form a brace and support my spine.	
I understand the role of my tranversus abdominis and lumbar multifidus muscles.	
I know how to move my pelvis in order to control the position of my low back.	
I know how to perform an abdominal brace on demand.	
I understand that core stabilization exercises are not about strength; they're about getting my muscles to work in sequence.	

Score 0-25

Knowing how to use your muscles to support and stabilize your spine is key to achieving a pain-free, functional back. When you limit your movement and physical activity because of back pain, you often also lose your ability to properly use your muscles to support and stabilize your spine.

The good news is that, with practice, it is a skill that can be relearned again. Use the movement patterns and exercise examples in Part 3 of this book to familiarize yourself again with how to use these muscles to brace your spine and place it in its optimum pain-free position.

Score 26-45

You have a good understanding of the role of movement and postural patterns in supporting and stabilizing your spine. What you need is to organize your exercise program to support your activities of daily living.

Knowing which particular exercise will support and stabilize your spine in which particular activity will give you the confidence to perform your usual tasks without fear of aggravating your low back pain symptoms.

Score 46+

Congratulations, you know how to use your muscles to position your spine in its pain-free, neutral position! Now, the key for you is consistency. Apply this skill set to your daily activities to minimize re-injury or recurrence of low back pain symptoms. You're on your way to achieving a pain-free functional back!

Hurdle #4. Compliance

Have you ever bought a piece of fancy hundred-dollar exercise equipment only for that equipment to gather dust in a corner after the first few weeks of using it?

I have. More than a couple of times. And, if you're being honest, you might have bought one of those pieces of equipment as well. And barely used it.

The same is true with an exercise program - it is hard to stay committed and see it through to its completion.

Here's what happens:

You enroll yourself in a back program; be it with a physical/physiotherapist, a chiropractor, a Yoga instructor, a posture or movement specialist, a back specialist, etc.

Just prior to starting, you were full of hope and anticipation of what you will accomplish with the program you enrolled yourself in. You start envisioning a better and healthier version of yourself.

Then you begin executing the necessary steps on your way to your envisioned future healthy self.

You start doing the different exercises and movement patterns introduced to you. These are new techniques and patterns that your body is not accustomed to. This is when you realize that it takes effort to change old unhealthy habits and adopt new paradigms of healthy living.

You start saying to yourself, "*This is hard.*"

But you keep on.

Then you slowly enter a dark but inviting alleyway in your mind by telling yourself, "*I don't have time right now, I'll do it later.*"

Or "*Not today, maybe tomorrow.*"

You start self-negotiating.

Until you finally admit to yourself, "*I suck at this. I quit.*"

Seth Godin, an American author, and former internet business executive, wrote a book and called this stage, "The Dip". Psychologists call it "The Valley of Despair".

This is the point where most people give up on their back program; unable to achieve their envisioned future healthy self.

Why?

Because it is hard to win a battle by yourself. Alone.

You need to enlist another person/other people to hold you accountable for the goals you set for yourself. Somebody who will hold your feet to the fire if you don't get up and move.

Human beings are social beings. We answer to others, sometimes more than to ourselves.

Left to our own volition and if given a choice, we would rather sit on the couch, munch potato chips, and binge-watch Netflix.

Your compliance and success with a back exercise program can be significantly increased by having another person hold you accountable when you're slipping down "The Dip". An accountability partner is able to perceive what you can't see when blind spots and weaknesses block your vision of your future self. And we all have blind spots.

That is why I built in an accountability component to the program, *Back Pain Unlocked System™*. It is to ensure we prompt people lagging behind in their exercises long before they slide down the valley of despair.

In this book, I discuss several strategies for keeping yourself committed and accountable.

For now, see how much accountability help you need by doing the assessment below.

Master the *Back Pain Unlocked System*™

Before we proceed with the rest of the book, let's review your ability to comply and stay consistent with your back program at home.

Below, rate yourself on a scale from 1 - 10 on how accurate the statements are—1 means "not accurate at all," and 10 means "most accurate."

Once you've rated yourself for each statement, total up your scores and then use the Answer Key to determine your next steps.

Self-Assessment Statement	Self-Rating
I'm able to stick with my exercise program through its completion.	
I don't have any problems staying consistent with my exercise schedule.	
I don't need reminders or external prompts to perform my exercises.	
I finish my exercises, no matter how challenging. I don't easily give up.	
I have an accountability partner who gives me cues to action in case I slide down the "Dip" or the "Valley of Despair".	
I have a working system to track my progress toward my physical activity goals.	

Score 0-29

You don't have to battle chronic low back alone. In fact, you shouldn't. Many people fail in their back programs, not because they lack the resolve to complete the program. They just don't have the proper support in place to point them in the right direction or to encourage them in case the going gets tough.

You need people in your corner helping you see your blind spots. You need partners giving you cues to action in case you fall off your back program.

Chronic low back pain can be an isolating experience, but your journey to recovery does not have to be.

Enlist people to help you in your back program. Identify people who can hold you accountable to your expressed exercise commitments and goals. Asking for help is not a sign of weakness. On the contrary, it takes courage, inner strength, and self-awareness to do so.

Score 30-44

Knowing isn't doing. You may be aware of what you need to do, but doing it consistently is a different thing. Having accountability prompts and cues to action can go a long way toward ensuring your success.

Create an accountability system to support your goal of achieving a pain-free functional back. Chronic low back pain does not happen in an instant. It took a while to develop from an acute episode to a prolonged pain experience. An accountability system will help you overcome the different hurdles along the way in your journey to recovery.

Score 45+

You are on your way to recovery! You are resolved to succeed in your back program, and you have a good accountability system and support to ensure your compliance and commitment to your goals. Use the examples of cognitive-behavioral tools and physical activities in Part 3 of this book to break free from the grip of chronic low back pain.

KEY CHAPTER TAKEAWAYS

- **Hurdle #1. Mind Matters**
  Pain is not just a physical sensation; it is a multidimensional experience. There are emotional, cognitive, behavioral, and social components to the pain experience. How you feel about your

pain, what you think about your pain, and how you perceive your well-being in relation to your experience of pain play a role in how you recover from chronic low back pain.

- **Hurdle #2. Lack of Clarity**
  Begin with the end in mind and let your goals inform the details of your exercise program. Your back exercise program has more power and efficacy if you know why you do what you do. It is helpful to have a road map to guide your journey of recovery and to reference when you are lost in the details.

- **Hurdle #3. Mastering Movement**
  Unlearning faulty postural habits and movement patterns while adopting correct and healthy ones can be a difficult process. But just like with any other skill, it can be learned. The result will be totally worth it. That is the key to preventing a frequent recurrence of your back pain and achieving a functional back. That is how you take your power back.

- **Hurdle #4. Compliance**
  Keeping and staying on course with any exercise program is hard. Recognize that human beings are social beings. Having another person hold you accountable for sticking with your back program will increase your likelihood of seeing your goals through completion.

Chapter 5

To Get Results, Untangle the Complexity

"Our life is frittered away by detail… simplify, simplify, simplify."

HENRY DAVID THOREAU

If chronic low back pain is a multifactorial and multidimensional experience, why is your current back program not addressing all the components involved?

The answer to that question holds the key to why most programs meant to address chronic low back pain do not work, and why the *Back Pain Unlocked System™* does.

Most back programs, including the ones you may have tried that didn't work, follow the old but still dominant practice of healthcare professionals in the western world - the "biomedical model." The biomedical model of health is the model of disability, purely focused in terms of biological or physical factors and excludes psychological, environmental, and social influences.

In this model, each illness has one underlying biological or physical cause, and once that cause is removed, the patient will be healthy again. What you think, believe, feel, or perceive, including the social factors informing your current pain experience are irrelevant to your back pain.

That is how your doctor ends up prescribing you with pain medications, injections, or surgery. That is how your physical/ physiotherapist ends up prescribing you with stretching and core strengthening exercises. Or your chiropractor ends up manipulating your spine. Or your acupuncturist sticking a needle into your skin. And I could go on and on with other treatment modalities and interventions focused solely on the physical component of your chronic low back pain.

But I wouldn't. By now you already know that addressing the physical component alone, though a critical part of a back program and surely included in the *Back Pain Unlocked System™*, is not sufficient if your goal is to achieve a pain-free functional back.

The *Back Pain Unlocked System™* follows the "biopsychosocial model" which is a multifactorial and integrative model that addresses the biological, psychological, and social components of your back pain experience. **You are a whole body, not a body part.** Like a three-legged stool, each leg is necessary and supports the other.

Back Pain Unlocked System™

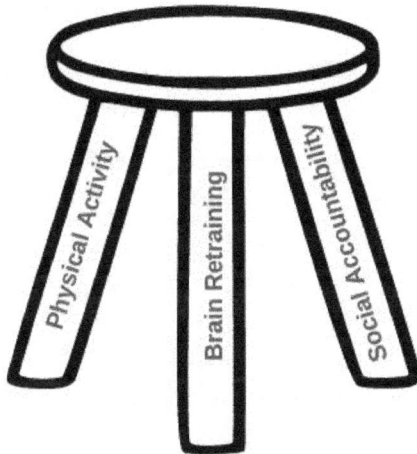

Figure 1. Addressing all three components of the chronic low back pain experience.

In later chapters, we'll explore each component of the *Back Pain Unlocked System™*. For now, let me tell you what the one thing to focus on that will give you a quick win while experiencing for yourself the power of the *Back Pain Unlocked System™* when applied.

Directional Preference

Have you noticed that certain positions or movements aggravate your back pain while doing the opposite relieves the symptoms? Do you refrain from certain activities for fear of aggravating your back pain?

If your pain is better or worse, depending on the position you are in, it means that your body prefers to be placed in certain positions for relief. If repeated weight-bearing or loading in a certain direction aggravates your pain, try repeated weight-bearing or loading in the opposite direction.

For example, does your back feel better when:

- You sleep on your stomach? Or when you sleep on your back with your knees or legs supported?

- You sit up tall? Or when you sit slouched forward?

- You lean forward on the sink to brush your teeth? Or when you lean back when gargling mouthwash?

- You lean forward on the grocery cart for support? Or when you stand up straight to push the grocery cart?

- You walk uphill? Or when you walk downhill?

Notice that these patterns are devoid of your diagnoses, i.e., degenerative disc disease, stenosis, bulging or herniated disc, etc. The reason is that your direction preference is movement-based, not diagnosis-based.

Now, once you determine your directional preference, combine your dynamic stabilization exercises (physical component) with guided visualization (psychological component) to overcome your learned bias of avoiding activities that may historically have caused pain. Tie the entire program with cues to action (social component) to help you be consistent not just with the exercises, but in applying the principles of proper body mechanics and back care.

You have just created your own comprehensive back program (for more details, see Part 3). You've addressed the different components and factors contributing to your chronic low back pain.

In 2008, a systematic review of randomized controlled trials was conducted to investigate the effectiveness of a biopsychosocial approach to the management of chronic low back pain. To compare the results, all the studies reviewed included measurements of both pain intensity and disability.[1]

The researchers compared different treatments and looked at how well they worked. One treatment was exercise alone (physical component), one was cognitive-behavioral therapy alone (psychosocial component), one was the usual care, and the last group had no treatment at all.

The study found strong evidence and supports the use of all three components as most effective in the treatment of chronic low back pain.

Let scientific research and evidence-based information help you in your decision to treat chronic low back pain.

If your goal is to achieve a pain-free functional back, let the *Back Pain Unlocked System*™ be your guide.

KEY CHAPTER TAKEAWAYS

- The old medical practice in Western medicine is deeply entrenched in the biomedical model. This model postulates that all disease is a product of biological or physical defects, devoid of psychological or social influences. That is how healthcare practitioners end up prescribing one-dimensional physical solutions, i.e., pain pill, steroid injection, surgery, exercise, or spinal manipulation, etc.

- Current research and evidence-based information support the effectiveness of using the biopsychosocial model, emphasizing patient-centered care and integrative medicine. You are a whole body, not a body part. This model accounts in its framework for the behavioral, psychological, and social dimensions of illness.

- For a back program to be effective and achieve long-term success, it needs to be comprehensive, addressing the different components of the pain experience.

Chapter 6

The Problem with Comprehensive Back Programs

*"Knowing what to do and not doing it
is the same as not knowing what to do."*

ROBIN SHARMA

Over and over, I've seen how effective comprehensive back programs like the *Back Pain Unlocked System*™ are in helping people break free from the grip of chronic low back pain.

But there's a fundamental problem with comprehensive back programs, which we will explore here.

Many people have tried addressing the different factors and components that contribute to their pain experience but have failed to achieve a pain-free functional back. The specific reason for their failure is the topic of this chapter.

Put simply, comprehensive back programs like the *Back Pain Unlocked System*™, require a significant personal investment.

If you don't apply yourself fully, the system, no matter how sound and effective as a means of achieving your goal, will not work.

It takes time, energy, and commitment to stay the course. You need to be open to learning, both with your mind and body. You need to be accountable not just for achieving your goal but, more importantly, for undergoing the mental and physical process required to adopt a new health paradigm.

People will have opinions about what you're trying to achieve. People close to you, full of good intent but possibly lacking in evidence-based information, will question your decisions. Pharmaceutical companies will only be too happy to offer you a pill to numb the pain. After all, there is money in disease, not health. Medical and surgical companies will gladly offer you a shot or a slice of your back.

For over 80 years, "disease management and rest" has dominated medicine in the United States.[1] It is hard to go against that heavy tide of healthcare culture.

So, if this is the reality, and it is, why am I such a proponent of using a comprehensive back program?

Well, it's quite simple, actually:

Most people, including healthcare providers, are doing it wrong.

Just teaching people suffering from chronic low back pain about the need to address the different components of the pain experience without providing them with the tools to succeed is not enough.

In the current healthcare environment we operate in, healthcare dollars are mostly being managed by insurance companies. They control the cost and balance the fiscal equation in either of two ways:

1. By putting limits on beneficiary coverages, i.e., high insurance copay, a limited number of visits allowed, etc.

2. By decreasing reimbursement for healthcare services rendered, i.e., decreasing payment to doctors, physical therapists, etc.

To check the authenticity of those statements, simply ask, "When was the last time your healthcare provider spent a good hour educating and providing you with the tools you need to succeed?"

Remember, you are the most important member of the recovery team.

If you are not provided with the education and the tools to succeed, how can you succeed?

That's the key difference here.

The #1 problem with comprehensive back programs is that it takes time, energy, and resources that the current fiscal environment of our healthcare system is not designed to provide. I wrote **Back Pain Unlocked** to provide you with the education and tools you need to succeed in your own journey to recovery.

In the next chapters, we'll explore the entire *Back Pain Unlocked System*™ for achieving a pain-free functional back. If you get nothing else from this book, please remember that you need a comprehensive back program to succeed. Not piecemeal information gathered from well-meaning friends or the internet. Or a hodgepodge of tools duct-taped to look like a back brace for your biopsychosocial needs.

KEY CHAPTER TAKEAWAYS

- A comprehensive back program, not one particular method, technique, or equipment, is the most effective way to treat chronic low back pain.

- The current fiscal environment of our healthcare system does not support a comprehensive back program.

- You are the most important member of the recovery team.

Part 2

BACK PAIN *UNLOCKED* *(BPU) SYSTEM*™

Chapter 7

How Your Back Looks Inside Out

"Your inner strength is your outer foundation."

-ALLAN RUFUS

Essential to the success of the *Back Pain Unlocked System*™ is having a clear-headed understanding of the structural strength inherent in the human spine. I find that many people come to me with perceived notions of how weak their backs are:

1. My doctor told me I have an "old man's back".

2. My X-ray or MRI is the worst my doctor has ever seen.

3. My back is "out of alignment" and needs to be put back in place.

4. My family has a history of arthritis and bad backs.

5. My core is so weak I need a back brace to support my spine.

Without a clear mental picture of how your back looks inside out, these common and popular myths about back pain can easily cloud your objectivity in the way you regard the strength of your spine.

Unproven and misleading ideas result in uncertainty and stress. In turn, the uncertainty and stress result in increased sensitivity to perceived threat or fear associated with your chronic low back pain.

So, how will you counter this vicious cycle?

By dispelling the myths and educating yourself on the inherent strength of your back.

Let's get started…

Imagine building a tower using Lego™ blocks stacked on top of the other. Our spine is designed the same way. Blocks of bone, called *vertebral bodies,* are stacked on top of the other. These blocks of bone start from the neck all the way down to the lower back to form the backbone or spine.

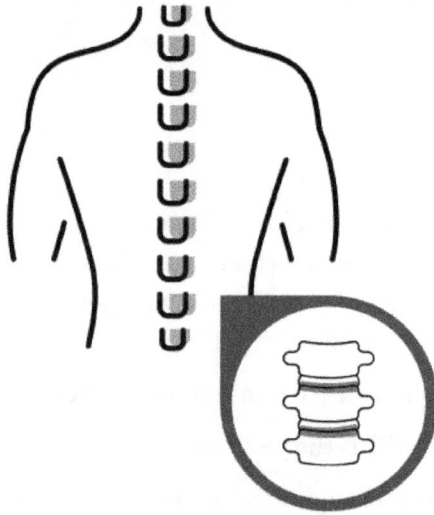

Figure 1. Vertebral spine and vertebral body

Now, picture placing a sponge in between each of those blocks of bone. The sponge placed in between the vertebral bodies allows for some freedom of movement between the stack of bones, as well as absorbing the weight and force transmitted through the spine. These sponges placed in between the blocks of bones are called *vertebral discs*.

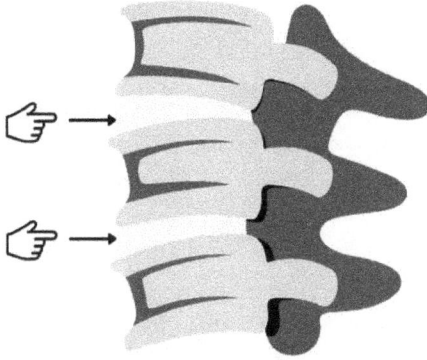

Figure 2. Vertebral disc

The vertebral discs are composed of soft gelatinous cartilage material in the center, enclosed in an outer casing of tough fibrous cartilage.

Unlike the muscles and organs of our bodies, the intervertebral disc is *a*vascular; meaning there is no blood flowing in and out of the disc.

The only way it gets nutrition and oxygen is through movement. When we move, blood flow increases to the periphery of the disc, which provides more nutrients and oxygen for healing. The movement also takes away chemicals caused by injury or age changes which can cause pain.

To add stability to this stack of bones, the blocks of bone have "scaffold-ings" in the back to help stabilize the weight of the tower. The areas of the scaffolding that meet are called *facet joints*.

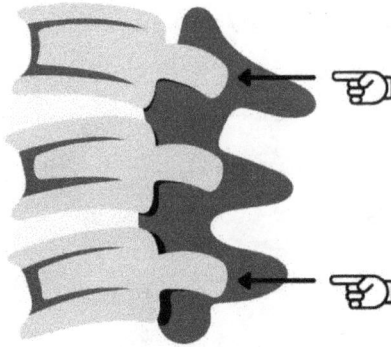

Figure 3. Facet joints

The facet joints are critical in that not only do they provide added stability to the spine, but they also control motion between each individual vertebral body. Because of these two opposing, yet complementing roles, the facet joints are subject to injury or wear and tear (arthritic) changes.

Another important role of the spine is to protect the spinal cord and nerves that act as the information highway between the body and the brain. This highway transmits both motor and sensory messages, including pain, up and down the body and the brain.

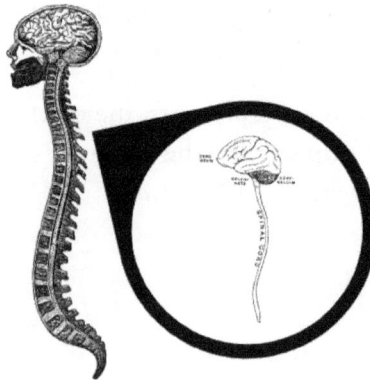

Figure 4. Spinal cord

The area where the nerve exits through the hole between the vertebrae is called the inter*vertebral foramen.* Over time, these holes may develop bony overgrowths, narrowing the space for the nerve roots to exit.

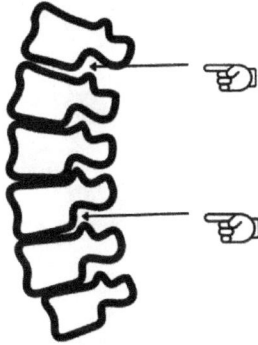

Figure 5. Intervertebral foramen

So, how does our body prevent these blocks of bone from collapsing?

Our body has two soft tissue structures that prevent our spine from collapsing.

The first soft tissue system that supports the spine is the ligaments. *Ligaments* are like duct tape sticking to the bones. These are bands of tough elastic tissue connecting bone to bone, holding the spine together, and limiting excessive movement between vertebrae to prevent injuries.

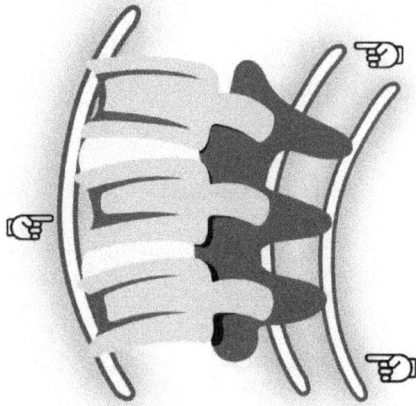

Figure 6. Ligaments connecting the spine

The second soft tissue system structure supporting our spine is the *muscles*. Imagine your spine like a mast on a ship. The muscles that attach to the spine are the ropes that support the mast and prevent it from becoming unstable and collapsing. As you can imagine, if the supporting muscles are weak or imbalanced, it'll cause the spine to be unstable and experience stress or pain. Weak muscles will cause the "mast" to sag or collapse.

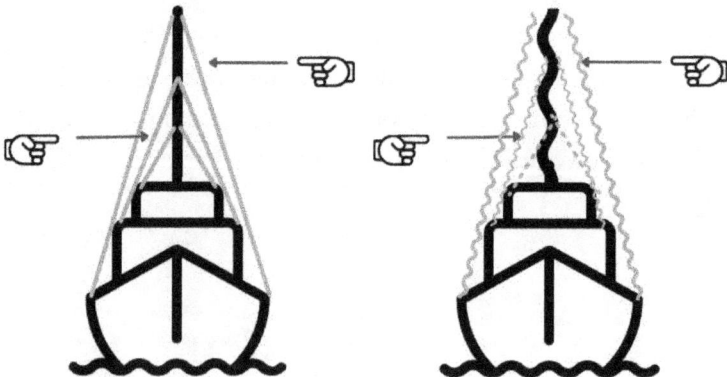

Figure 7. Strong vs. weak back muscles supporting the length of your spine.

In the muscular system supporting the spine, there are short muscles that support and control motion from one vertebra to the adjacent vertebra. One of these small, yet powerful muscles is called the *multifidus*. Think of your multifidus muscle as a strong chain linking and stabilizing one vertebral body to the next.

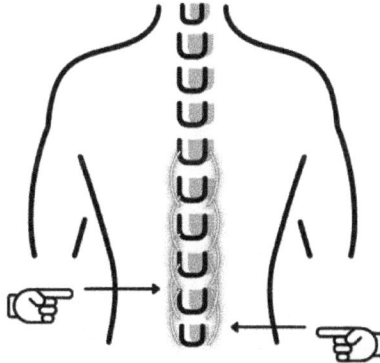

Figure 8. Multifidus muscles

There are also longer muscles that attach to multiple vertebrae, supporting the length of the spine. These muscles are called *erector spinae*. They ran vertically on each side of the spine, extending and stabilizing the entire vertebral column. Think of your erector spinae muscles like guy wires supporting a tall tower.

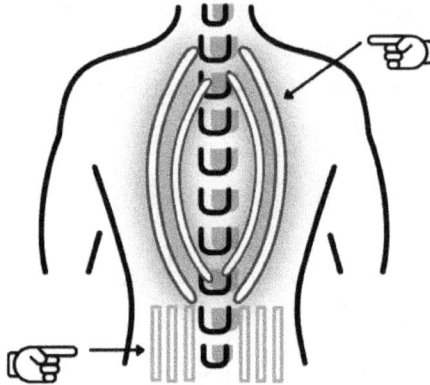

Figure 9. Erector spinae (long muscles) and quadratus lumborum (thick muscles).

Additionally, there are also thick muscles on the front, sides, and back of the spine that act as a brace, further supporting the back. These muscles are sometimes called your core or "corset muscles" as they are responsible for bracing your spine in anticipation of your body moving. The primary "corset" muscles are composed of your transversus abdominis, internal and external obliques, and the superficial rectus abdominis, and the quadratus lumborum in the back.

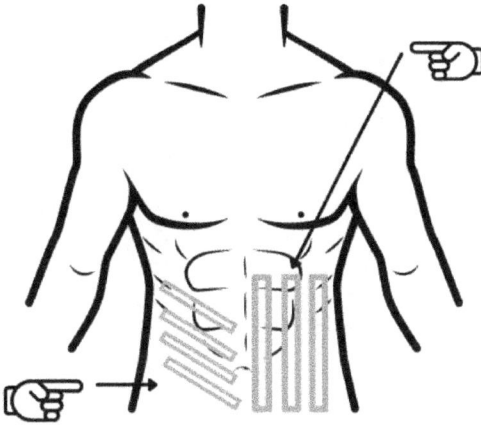

Figure 10. Core ("corset") muscles

Don't worry about memorizing the names of these muscles. What is more important is knowing how to use them.

Because of the length of the spine, it would take a lot of energy for those muscles to stabilize it from the neck all the way down to the low back. Our body solves this problem by creating curves, dispersing the weight and forces through opposing curves in the spine instead of bearing the weight, and forces straight up and down through the length of the spine.

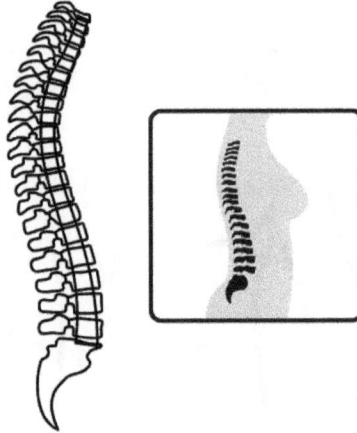

Figure 11. Normal spine curvature

As you can see, your spine is inherently strong. It has multiple structures that support and prevent the tower of vertebral bones from collapsing.

Now that you have a clear mental picture of the inherent strength of your spine, devoid of myths and hazy ideas, you will not struggle with the physical activity component of the *Back Pain Unlocked System™*.

You are now armed with the knowledge that, unless you're pulling or pushing an 18-wheel Mack truck, the regular exercises, and daily activities you do will not harm you.

(By the way, in May 2020, Men's Health magazine reported that a guy named Brian Shaw expanded his home workout to include pulling his 8,000- lbs. truck hand-over-hand up his inclined driveway!)

But what if you have been diagnosed with any of the following conditions?

- Bulging disc
- Herniated disc

- Spinal stenosis

- Vertebral stenosis

- Slipped disc

- Slipped vertebra

- Degenerative disc disease

These diagnoses, frequently seen in medical imaging results (X-rays, MRIs, CT scans, etc.) scare patients and cause stress and anxiety. And for good reason; albeit for a reason that might surprise you.

People are naturally afraid of things they don't understand. It threatens their sense of self, their security, their very existence. Not knowing the meaning of the diagnosis on your medical imaging can produce an unpleasant feeling triggered by the perception of danger, whether real or imagined.

How will you counter that fear?

Once again, by letting data and evidence based information inform your thoughts and behavior toward these diagnoses.

What medical imaging tells us about back pain:

When seeing a doctor for back pain, it's common for the doctor to order an imaging test. These tests usually show some sort of abnormality, disease, or injury. But just because they found something on your X-ray or MRI, or scan does not mean you have to be limited in what you can do or how much pain you feel.

It is possible to have something wrong on your back and not know it.

The opposite is also true - it is possible you are experiencing back pain, yet your medical imaging results will not show any significant findings.

Do not let your medical imaging results scare you. Find out what they mean so that you can put the information into perspective and make an informed decision on how to manage your pain.

worn down due to aging, there can be more space for nerves at risk of being impinged on by bone spurs (osteophytes).

This is called "degenerative" because it means our spine is deteriorating with time — as with the rest of our body.

Age-related changes, including degenerative disc disease, do not have a direct correlation with back pain. If it is, everyone over the age of 20 should have back pain and no one below 20 should have back pain.

The imaging pictures show changes that happen with age. This does not mean you have to be in pain or be limited in what you can do.

It can be scary to hear your doctor say that you have a slipped vertebra, a bulging disc, a herniated disc, spinal stenosis, or degenerative disc disease and not know what it means for the future of your health and function.

The truth is that there is no relationship between what the medical imaging pictures show and how you feel or function.

Dr. David Hanscom, a renowned orthopedic spinal deformity surgeon and author of Back in Control: A Surgeon's Roadmap Out of Chronic Pain[5], has this to say about imaging results and surgery:

"We generally don't know where back pain comes from exactly. We do know very clearly that disc degeneration has nothing to do with back pain. So, conditions such as arthritis, bone spurs, bulging, herniated, "slipped" or ruptured discs are rarely the underlying cause of the problem.

This is where spinal surgery – probably about 70 percent of it should not be done. Yet in America we are probably doing between 400,000 and half a million spinal fusions a year – with a success rate of only about 22-24 percent.

Medical imaging results are not an accurate predictor of pain. Many people who suffer from severe pain have completely normal MRIs, and many people who have abnormal MRI results experience no pain at all.

So, where is the pain coming from?

I'm glad you asked! Let's turn to the next chapter to learn some more.

KEY CHAPTER TAKEAWAYS

- Having a clear understanding of the anatomical and structural strength inherent in your spine will help you overcome your fear of movement or physical activities.

- Do not let your medical imaging results scare you. While the pictures and diagnoses seen in your medical imaging (MRI, X-ray, scans) are useful for ruling out important things like tumors and disease pathology, they are not good at predicting, explaining, or treating pain conditions or dysfunction.

- Let data and evidence-based information inform your thoughts and behavior toward these diagnoses.

Chapter 8

Where Pain Is Coming From

"Pain is real. But so is hope."

ANONYMOUS

So, if your back is inherently strong and your medical imaging results do not have a direct correlation to your pain and dysfunction, where is your pain coming from then?

That is the same question asked by a group of researchers and clinicians focused on the study of the science of pain. What they found out was both enlightening and instructive for people suffering from chronic low back pain - the more you know and understand about pain and the more you know what to do about it, the less you will experience pain.[1-2]

Neuroscience and the BioPsychoSocial Model

Since pain interacts with many different things, to better understand pain, we need to use a model that takes into account the different factors contributing to pain.

The biopsychosocial model serves us well as it looks at what has gone wrong with the body and brain as well as how the illness is lived. It looks not only at the disease or injury, but also takes into account any psychological or social factors that may influence our perception of pain.[3]

The biopsychosocial approach to treating back pain is based on an understanding that it's not just about getting the injury or disease healed, but also making sure that people can continue to function and have a good quality of life.[4]

Get acquainted with your living alarm system.

There are a lot of nerves in your body. If connected from end to end, those nerves would extend up to 45 miles. This network of nerves connects all of your body parts to form the superhighway of your body's alarm system.[5]

Think of your body's alarm system as kind of like the high striker tower (sometimes called strongman game) you often would see at state fairs.

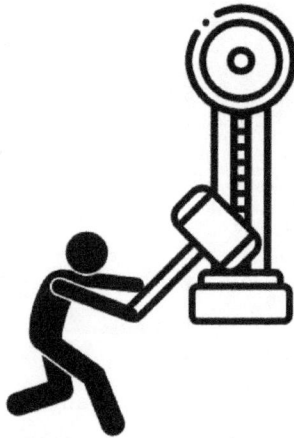

Figure 1. High Striker Tower, the body's living alarm system.

Imagine that the *plate* a player will strike on is your back.

The *alarm* at the top of the tower is your brain.

The *lever* that connects the plate and the alarm is your superhighway of nerves.

In most cases, your body will respond to a back injury by sending signals of pain from the nerve endings located in your back (the plate) through the network of nerves (the lever) up to your brain (the alarm bell). This message goes into your consciousness for you to know something is wrong with your back.

As soon as pain is felt and action has been taken, the alarm system calms down, and the lever will return to its resting level. The initial injury passed as the player took the hammer off the plate of the high striker tower. After all, the player will have to pick up the hammer off the plate, right?

So where is the pain coming from again, you asked?

Pain is an output of your brain!

Pain is your brain's opinion of how much danger you are in. When you think that something is dangerous, your brain produces pain so it can protect you.[6]

The alarm bell (your brain) will ring to indicate that somebody or something has struck, or is about to strike, the plate (your back)!

Chronic low back pain

What happens in chronic low back pain is that the lever (your nerves) sometimes gets stuck and remains elevated near the alarm (your brain).

In this state, it doesn't take much "striking" to make the alarm bell ring, sending off danger messages to your consciousness.

Since you first became conscious of the pain, you've noticed that even your usual tasks or your usual amount of stress exacerbate your back pain.[7]

Your body's alarm system has become extra sensitive to protect you - the lever is stuck too close to the alarm.[8-9]

How would you know if your alarm system is being extra sensitive?"

Here are some signs that your alarm system could be extra sensitive:

- You notice that you have limited or restricted your physical activities.
- You have stopped taking part in activities you used to do with ease.
- You are afraid to move your back.
- You are sensitive to pressure around your back.
- You asked your doctor for medications to help calm your nerves.

Why would this alarm system remain sensitive?

Some people have other psychosocial factors and stressors that make them susceptible to experiencing continuing pain. The brain chooses to keep the alarm system on high alert, so the person doesn't get hurt again. Then they can feel safe.

Psychosocial factors and stressors that can prolong the sensitivity of your alarm system can include:

- **Anxiety and depression** can make you feel like your pain will never go away. There are other problems that come with anxiety and depression, like chronic fatigue and insomnia, which make it harder to recover from injury and get better.
- **Fear of activities** that may hurt your back or make it worse. This can include fear of getting out of bed, bending over to pick up something you dropped on the floor or wearing anything tight around your waistline. Inactivity or decreased mobility prolongs back pain, not hastens its healing.
- **Pain catastrophizing** is a fairly common issue in which a person thinks their pain will never end and becomes frightened by the

idea of doing anything to make it better. A study done in 2000 has shown that fear of injury, re-injury, and fear of movement or exercises will keep the alarm system turned on.[10]

- **Past treatment experience**. If you have found relief from treatment with a certain doctor, physical/physiotherapist, or chiropractor, then the experience will make you feel more confident about your treatment outcome. Likewise, if you have a history of unsuccessful treatments without relief from symptoms, this might lead to an increased level of negative expectations which can worsen the symptoms.

- **Stress.** Many things can cause stress, from the demands of a job, change in relationship status, to the loss of a loved one. If your brain continues to have worries and concerns from chronic or repeated stress, your alarm system will continue to be on high alert, a condition called *stress-induced hyperalgesia*.[11]

For people who experience back pain for an extended period of time (more than 12 weeks), there is evidence suggesting they have developed changes in their brain as well as physical injury. This explains why many patients with back injuries continue to feel pain even when their acute injury has healed. They have developed a psychological response to the initial event.[12]

No, the pain is not all in your head.

On the contrary, when you are feeling pain, remember that it is a multidimensional experience. There are sensory, emotional, and cognitive components to pain - or the way it feels, how you feel about it, and how you perceive your well-being in relation to your experience of pain.

Your pain is real. I am not going to tell you that everything is just fine.

But your pain is not an indicator of physical damage in your body. And I am confident you will get better.

A conversation I recently had with one of my patients illustrates this concept succinctly:

She started by telling me, "My dad has been battling lung cancer for 4 years now and I have been his primary caregiver for the past three years."

"One time, I helped dad get up from the bed to transfer to his wheelchair. As soon as I leaned back to turn, I felt a sharp, excruciating pain in my low back."

"This was over a year ago. I knew I should have taken the time to treat my back pain. But who has the time to exercise when you have a family to feed and an ailing father to care for?"

"I don't know if I was feeling guilty to take the time off to care for myself, or if I was too embarrassed to ask for help."

"I didn't know my social situation and even my mental and emotional state all contributed to my continuing back pain. And to think I almost elected to have surgery last week."

"I knew I could do something about my back pain. I knew I could come out victorious!"

As she leaves my office, I hear her saying those words. She was talking to herself, not to me.

She is finally in charge.

KEY CHAPTER TAKEAWAYS

- Pain is an output of your brain. It is your brain's opinion of how much danger you are in. When you think that something is dangerous, your brain produces pain so it can protect you.

- Your beliefs, behavior, emotions, attitude, stressors, and environment all inform your experience of pain and can cause your living alarm system to remain hypersensitive.

- Using cognitive-behavioral tools, you can reframe your brain's opinion of how much danger you are in and lower your alarm system's sensitivity.

Chapter 9

Putting It All Together

*"The secret of success in life is for a man to be
ready for his opportunity when it comes."*

BENJAMIN DISRAELI

In Chapter 7, you gained a foundational understanding of the different
structures supporting your back allowing its inherent strength. In Chapter
8, you learned about the neuroscience of pain and the different cognitive,
behavioral, and social factors informing your experience of pain.

**You now know more about your back and the science of
pain more than the next hundred people around you.**

In this chapter, we will break down the critical pieces of each of the three
components that need to be in place for you to achieve the outcome you
want.

Why is a comprehensive system more powerful and effective than any of the methods you've tried before? Because a system is more than just any one method, technique, procedure, or approach.

A quick dictionary search for the meaning of the word *system* gave me this definition:

system / **sis**-*tuh*m / *noun*

1. An ordered and comprehensive assemblage of facts, principles, or the like in a particular field of study or thought.

2. A coordinated body of methods or plan of procedure; organizational scheme.

What I'm sharing with you is a comprehensive set of methods and techniques I organized and developed for my patients. You now have it in your hands.

Let me share with you the Venn diagram of the *Back Pain Unlocked System*™ so you can have a 20,000-foot view of the critical pieces you need to achieve your goal of a pain-free functional back.

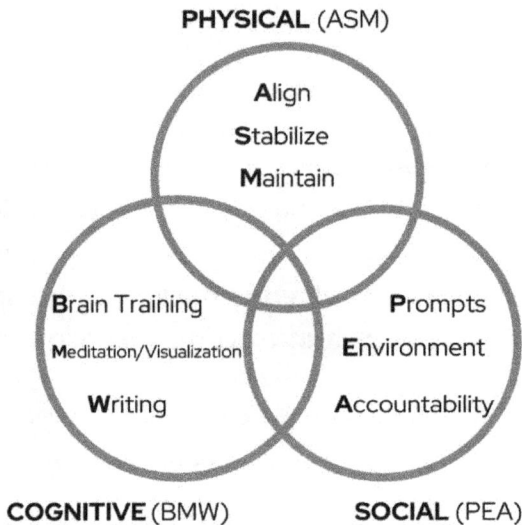

Figure 1. Back Pain Unlocked System™

All components overlap each other as each one is critical to the other. You can't resolve chronic low back pain with exercise alone. Or meditation alone. Or modifying your environment alone. Each component builds on the other to create a successful long-term result. Use this framework to your advantage.

Physical Component

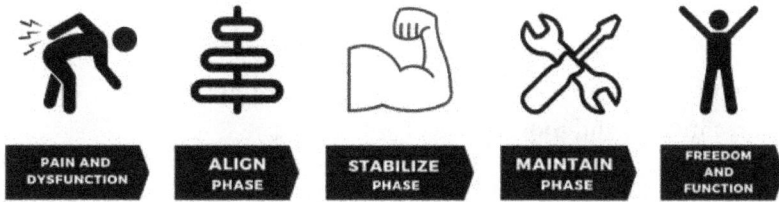

Figure 2. ASM Roadmap™

Not only is the *Back Pain Unlocked System™* comprehensive, it is also a logical and well-coordinated program.

You may have noticed in many back programs that the emphasis is on strengthening your core right from the get-go. You were taught that in order to fix your back pain, you have to strengthen your back and abdominal muscles. That is true. But that is placing the cart before the horse.

If all you need is a strong back to fix your back pain, then wouldn't that imply that people who are weak should have back pain and people who are strong should not have back pain?

This would mean that strong, weightlifting, bodybuilding athletes should not experience back pain. After all, these are some of the strongest groups of athletes in all sports.

But a study among young athletes in the sport of bodybuilding found that back pain was the most common complaint.[1]

Back pain injuries often occur due to improper execution of the techniques or lifting excessive weights.[2]

That is why the physical component of the *Back Pain Unlocked System*™ starts with ALIGN. Because when you start with strengthening exercises first, you will end up strengthening your back… in the wrong position.

A strong back in an incorrect position can only add to your back pain.

Starting with ALIGN teaches you to first achieve the optimum pain-free position of your spine, also called your "neutral spine position", using different techniques and movements of your pelvis.

You will learn how to move and control your pelvis. You will release the usual suspects of tight muscles in incessant states of spasm, holding your spine captive to incorrect or strained positions. You will learn about your back's direction preference or bias.

Once you find the optimum, pain-free position of your spine, then you move on to the STABILIZATION phase. Many people have the misconception that back stabilization exercises are meant to strengthen the back and core muscles. That is true. But again, that is placing the cart before the horse.

The value of back stabilization exercises is in training you on how to promote coordinated contractions of your back and core muscles. Back stabilization exercises are not about strength; they're about getting your muscles to work in proper sequence.[3] Muscle strength and endurance will be the result of those repetitions.

Once you've mastered the ALIGN and STABILIZATION phases of the *Back Pain Unlocked System*™, you will move on to the MAINTENANCE phase.

In the maintenance phase, you will apply the position and movement patterns you have learned from the first two phases into your activities of daily living.

Picking up a package from the floor?

Getting up from a low seat or toilet?

Sitting all day at work?

You will not have a problem in any of those situations; you'll know what to do in each one of those.

That is FREEDOM from pain and dysfunction.

Cognitive Component

As I have shared with you in the first chapter, properly executing the physical exercises with the wrong mental, emotional, or behavioral framework can still lead to failure. But once your mindset changes, everything on the outside will change along with it.

That is where brain retraining, writing, meditation, and guided visualization or graded motor imagery becomes indispensable.

Modern research tells us that chronic and recurring pain is caused by many triggers. The way we think and behave can affect how much pain we have and how often it recurs. Pain neuroscience has taught us that there is a connection between the brain and our physical pain sensations and that the brain has a significant influence on how we experience pain.

The cognitive component of The Back Pain Unlocked System™ gives you the tools to think differently about your relationship with pain. If retraining your thoughts and beliefs results in less worry, less anxiety, or increased expectation of a positive outcome, imagine what that would mean to your journey of recovery.

In his book, The Seven Habits of Highly Effective People, Stephen Covey said, *"All things are created twice. Vision is the first creation. For a house it's called the blueprint. For a life it's called a mission. For a day it's called a goal and a plan. For a parent it's called a belief in the unseen potential of a child.*

For all, it is the mental creation which always precedes the physical, or second creation."

Using the cognitive tools in the *Back Pain Unlocked System*™ will help you create a picture in your mind where you move without pain and limitation, your first creation. Your first creation in turn will help you to move in your physical environment without fear, pain, and limitation - your second creation.

If you don't believe in your mind that you can move without pain, you will have a hard time moving your physical body without pain. No matter how much exercise you do.

Use these cognitive tools to supercharge your back program.

Social Component

"No man or woman is an island."

The pain experience can be a lonely and isolating experience. Friends and family may empathize with you, but no other person feels what you are feeling right now. Your day-to-day struggle is real.

So, what about your support? Is it day-to-day as well?

Identify a specific person or several people who can give you action prompts for you to get back to your back program in case you start to slide down to "The Dip" or "The Valley of Despair".

Ensure that other people hold you accountable for the outcome you set for yourself. Human beings are inclined toward stasis, yet the outcome you desire requires change and growth. Left to our own devices, we often self-negotiate; struggling to achieve our goals without being held accountable by other people. Human beings are social beings - we sometimes do for others what we cannot do for ourselves.

Create a system of accountability where other people can provide you with *cues for action* to help you be compliant and consistent with your back program.

Also, create an environment that will support you to succeed. Sometimes it's as simple as changing the chair you often sit on that does not promote a good sitting posture. Or changing your habit of falling asleep on a couch that doesn't properly support your back. Sometimes, it is the more difficult decision of peeling yourself away from situations or people that add to your stress and anxiety.

Back in the introduction, I wrote that treating back pain at home is not easy or quick but is possible. Incorporating the different critical pieces I outlined for you in this chapter is what will make treating your back pain at home successful.

If you have tried different back programs before and failed to achieve long-term success, it is not your fault. You need tools more than just what fancy gadgets, equipment, or exercises can provide. I would highly recommend you follow the framework of the *Back Pain Unlocked System*™.

It'll likely change your life.

KEY CHAPTER TAKEAWAYS

- Your back exercise program not only has to be comprehensive, but it also needs to be logical and well-coordinated. If you start with strengthening exercises without first learning how to align your spine, you will strengthen your spine in the wrong position, causing more pain and recurrence of injury.

- Use cognitive-behavioral tools to retrain your brain and nervous system to lower its hypersensitivity to pain. Reframing your inner dialogue and your brain's opinion of the perceived or actual threat to your body will, in turn, give you the power to regulate your experience of pain.

- Having a system of accountability, appropriately utilizing support systems and tools, can significantly improve your chances of being consistent and compliant with your back program. The social component of a comprehensive back program is the glue that will ensure the success of your program.

Part 3

IMPLEMENTING THE BPU SYSTEM™

Chapter 10

Achieve Neutral Spine Position
(ALIGN Phase)

"Who you are tomorrow begins with what you do today."

— TIM FARGO

I always like to tell my patients that achieving a pain-free, neutral spine position is a lot like locating a comfortable neighborhood to live in, rather than searching for a specific address.

Many people get frustrated with how difficult it is to achieve a pain-free, neutral spine the way a lot of back programs teach them. That is because they were being taught to find a specific angle or position their spine needs to be in. But a pain-free, neutral spine needs to feel natural and comfortable, not rigid or tense.

You don't need to find a specific address. As long as you are in the neighborhood, you are good!

The goal of Back Pain Unlocked is not just to get rid of your back pain symptoms but for you to live with minimal limitations in mobility and function. Thus, achieving and maintaining optimum alignment of your spine is essential for the achievement of your goal.

If you've been experiencing low back pain symptoms for over three months or longer, you might have developed an aversion to certain movements or activities that seem to trigger pain, but are actually normal, healthy activities.[1-2]

One of the first movements people with chronic low back pain tend to limit is the movement of their pelvis. When you first hurt your back, rocking your pelvis forward or backward seemed to aggravate your pain. In fact, any movement around the area of your back seemed to cause more pain. To mitigate the initial back pain symptoms, you may have learned to minimize or limit the movement of your pelvis.

Over time, you have learned to not bend over from a standing position or pick up a package from the floor. You may have stopped walking or jogging, or even just sitting down for long periods of time.

With chronic pain, your brain tells you to be careful because it has learned that normal functions you used to perform with ease are now unsafe and dangerous activities. When you bend over to pick up a package from the floor, your brain produces pain signals to protect you from hurting yourself. When you walk, or jog, or sit down for longer periods of time, your brain produces pain as a form of protection. Your brain is being hyper-protective of you.

However, if this learned limitation of movement is extended over a period longer than the initial injury, this learned behavior will prolong your pain rather than help with your recovery.

Remember, pain is your brain's opinion of how much danger you are in, whether real or perceived.

Using the framework you learned in the *Back Pain Unlocked System*™, you have the tool and power to change that opinion.

Your brain can learn to be less hyper-protective by using a cognitive tool that elite athletes use. It is called Graded Motor Imagery. Use this tool to imagine yourself doing an activity you may have learned to be fearful of.

Cognitive Activity

1. Start in a sitting position.

2. Close your eyes and visualize yourself slowly rocking your pelvis forward and backward.

3. Using your imagination only, push your belly button as far forward as you can. Imagine pushing your pelvis all the way forward. Maintain this position while counting to five seconds.

4. Using your imagination only, now pull your belly button as far backwards as you can. Imagine pulling your pelvis all the way back. Maintain this position while counting to five seconds.

5. Using your imagination only, move back to your original position.

6. Any comfortable, pain-free position between positions #3 and #4 is your neutral spine position.

If you start to feel tense or anxious during this exercise, draw your attention to your breath and take a few slow deep breaths and ask yourself this question:

"Can the act of imagining yourself rocking your pelvis back and forth cause actual damage to your back?"

By asking this question, you give the conscious part of your brain the chance to overrule the unconscious part of your brain, where your learned behavior of limited movement lives.

Now close your eyes and repeat steps #1-5 by visualizing yourself comfortably rocking your pelvis back and forth until you don't feel tense or anxious performing the movement in your mind.

Once you feel comfortable visualizing yourself rocking your pelvis forward and backward, you can now move on to the physical component of the *Back Pain Unlocked System™*.

Physical Component

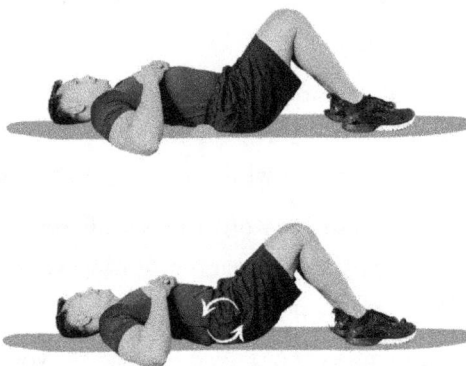

Figure 1. Lumbo-Pelvic Control

Lie down on a firm bed, exercise mat, or the floor if it's comfortable. When you perform pelvic rocking from this position, you're essentially taking the natural curve out of your lower back, flattening your back, then bringing it back to its pain-free neutral spine position.

1. Lie on your back with bent knees and the soles of your feet on the floor. In this position, the natural curve of your lumbar spine will lift the lower back slightly off the floor.

2. Exhale and slowly tilt your pelvis toward your head by engaging your abdominal muscles to pull your belly button back to your spine. As you do this, you'll feel your lower back pressing into the floor.

3. Maintain this position while counting to five seconds.

4. Return to your original position.

5. Do 10-15 reps.

Once you achieve mastery of this activity, progress to the next activity.

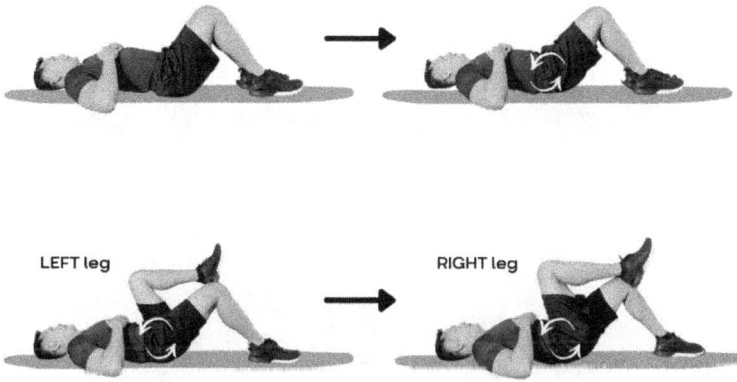

LEFT leg   RIGHT leg

Figure 2. Lumbo-Pelvic Control Progression #1

1. Lie on your back with bent knees and the soles of your feet on the floor. In this position, the natural curve of your lumbar spine will lift the lower back slightly off the floor.

2. Exhale and slowly tilt your pelvis toward your head by engaging your abdominal muscles to pull your belly button back to your spine. As you do this, you'll feel your lower back pressing into the floor.

3. Once you've engaged your abs and tilted your pelvis you will lift one foot up off the ground, bringing your knee in toward your chest.

4. Make sure that as you lift the knee toward your chest, your low back stays firmly on the ground. Touch that foot back down on the floor and raise the other knee in toward your chest.

5. Keep alternating legs, marching for 10-15 reps on each leg.

Note: This should be a controlled march that you can speed up as you become confident in your ability to keep your low back against the ground and your core braced.

Once you achieve mastery of this activity, progress to the next activity.

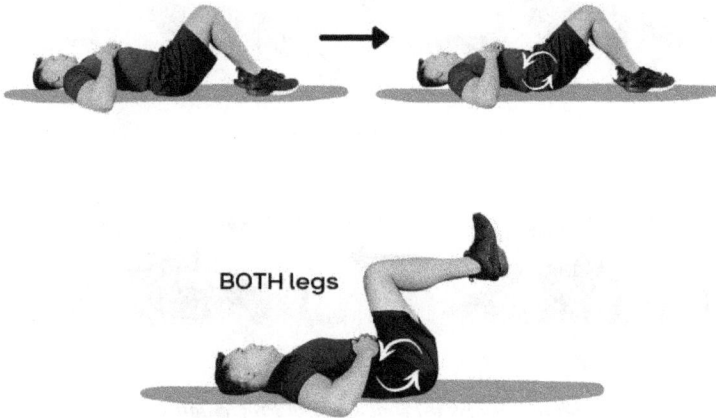

Figure 3. Lumbo-Pelvic Control Progression #2

1. Lie on your back with bent knees and the soles of your feet on the floor. In this position, the natural curve of your lumbar spine will lift the lower back slightly off the floor.

2. Exhale and slowly tilt your pelvis toward your head by engaging your abdominal muscles to pull your belly button back to your spine. As you do this, you'll feel your lower back pressing into the floor.

3. Lift both of your knees toward your chest. Move slowly and make sure to keep your low back against the ground as you lift both knees.

4. Slowly lower your feet down to the ground to release the contraction of your abdominal muscles.

Note: If at any point your abs aren't engaged and your low back isn't firmly pressed into the ground, pause and reset or regress the movement back to the march (Progression #1) until you are ready for the double knee tuck.

It is very important that you focus on quality movements and not just progressing as quickly as you can.

Direction Preference

Based on your back's direction preference (see Chapter 4), follow the directions below:

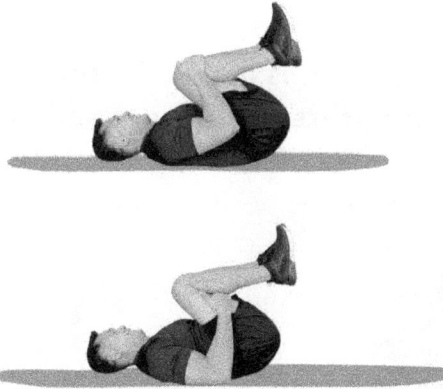

Alternate Position of Hands

Figure 4. Flexion Bias

To perform the supine low back flexion exercise, you must find a place to lie down on your back. The surface you lie upon should be supportive but still offer some comfort.

Performing the lumbar flexion exercise on your bed is not recommended if the mattress or cushion is too soft that your spine "sinks down" in the mattress or cushion during exercise.

1. Lie on your back.

2. Bend both knees up and put your feet flat on the ground.

3. Slowly bring both knees up towards your chest by grabbing your knees with your hands.

   (*Alternate Position*) If pressure on your knees causes knee pain, you can grab your thighs underneath your knees.

4. Gently pull your knees up close to your chest. Hold this position for 5 seconds.

5. Slowly allow your knees to lower back down to the starting position. Your feet should be flat on the floor and your knees should be bent.

6. Perform 10 repetitions.

Once you complete this activity without symptom aggravation, progress to the next activity.

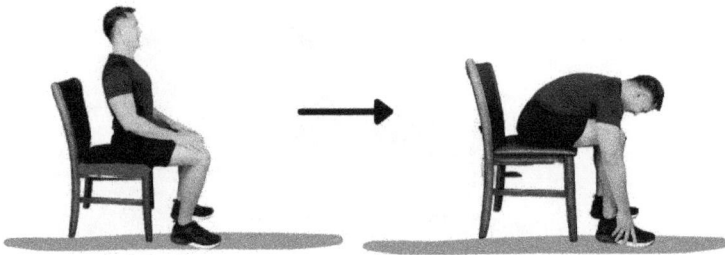

Figure 5. Flexion Bias Progression #1

1. Sit in a chair with your knees open and your feet on the floor.

2. Lean forward, bending at your low back.

3. Reach your hands down towards the floor and hold this position for two to five seconds.

4. Return to the starting position.

5. Repeat 5 times.

Once you complete this activity without symptom aggravation, progress to the next activity.

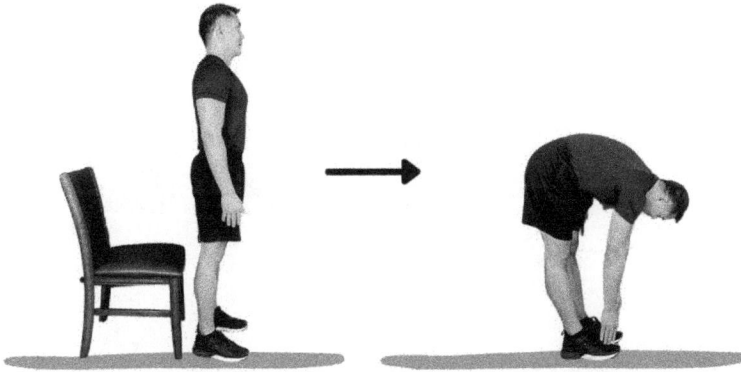

Figure 6. Flexion Bias Progression #2

1. Stand with your feet about shoulder-width apart.

2. Bend forward at the waist slowly.

3. Reach your hands down towards your feet as far as possible and hold this position for five seconds.

4. Return to the starting position.

5. Repeat 5 times.

Note: Remember to monitor your symptoms as you perform flexion exercises. If your symptoms improve, perform all 5-10 repetitions. If your symptoms worsen, reassess if your back has an extension bias/preference.

Do not continue stretching through lumbar flexion if your pain is worsening. If your pain improves, the low back flexion exercise can be performed several times per day.

What is the difference between the lumbo-pelvic control exercise and the flexion exercise?

Lumbo-pelvic control exercises are *active* exercises. You use the muscles attached to your pelvis, including your abdominals and hip muscles, to actively tilt your pelvis forward or backward.

Flexion exercises are *passive* exercises. You use your hands to bring your knees up to your chest to effect a stretch on your low back.

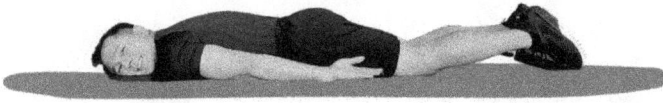

Figure 7. Extension Bias

If your symptoms decrease or go away altogether when you lean back or arch your back, your back condition likely has an extension bias.

1. Lie down on your stomach with your arms under your shoulders or down at your side.

2. Position your face down or turned to one side.

3. Take slow, deep breaths and relax.

4. Hold for 5 min.

Once you complete this activity without symptom aggravation, progress to the next activity.

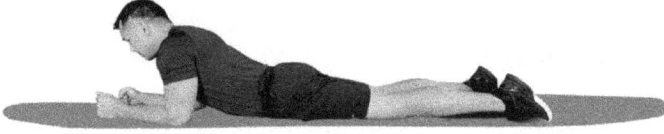

Figure 8. Extension Bias Progression #1

1. Lie down on your stomach and place your elbows under your shoulders so you are resting on your forearms.

2. Take slow, deep breaths and relax.

3. Hold for 1 minute then return to the original position.

4. Repeat 10 times

Once you complete this activity without symptom aggravation, progress to the next activity.

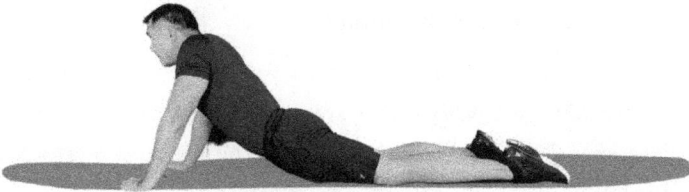

Figure 9. Progression #2

1. Lie down on your stomach and place your hands under your shoulders.

2. Slowly straighten elbows, keeping your lower body relaxed and your pelvis down on the floor while raising your back upwards as far as pain will allow.

3. Take slow, deep breaths and relax.

4. Hold for 1 minute.

5. Repeat 10 times.

Unlock and Stretch

There are certain muscles that often "lock-up" because of back pain. Either because of true adaptive muscle tightness or protective muscle tension, the tightness or tension on these muscles often makes it difficult to achieve a pain-free neutral spine.

Before jumping straight to a stretching exercise, remember the two reasons a muscle may "lock up":

1. *Protective muscle tension* – This is your muscle's protective mechanism. Your muscle reacts to pain by reflexively increasing its tension, sometimes referred to as muscle spasm, to protect the further movement of a painful body part. By stretching the muscle, you are effectively increasing its tension, further stimulating its protective mechanism (also called reflex inhibition).

   Muscles in this state will respond better to an unlocking technique, not a stretch technique.

2. *Adaptive muscle tightness* – This is your muscle's adaptive response to a prolonged position or state of contraction. For example, if you spend most of the day sitting, the muscles in front of your hips are adaptively shorter and tighter.

   Muscles in this state will respond to most stretching exercises you are familiar with.

I recommend that you start with the unlocking technique to first address the protective tension your muscles may have developed in response to your chronic low back pain. Once you've achieved mastery of this activity only then should you proceed with the stretching techniques.

Iliopsoas

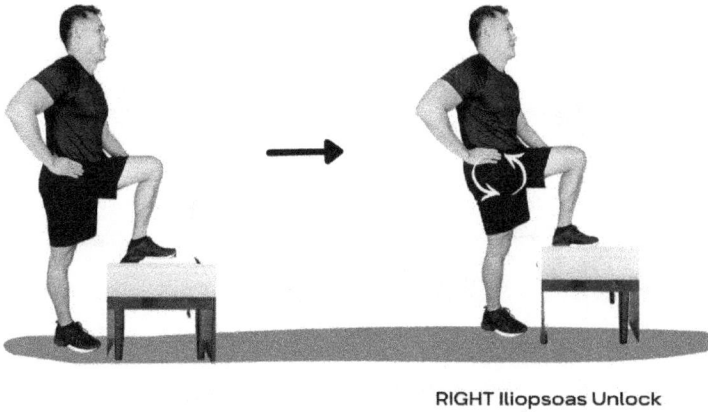

RIGHT Iliopsoas Unlock

Figure 10. Iliopsoas Unlock

1. While standing, place your left foot on top of a chair in front of you.

2. Stand upright and tilt your pelvis posteriorly, unlocking the iliopsoas muscle in front of your right hip.

3. Return your pelvis to its original position.

4. Repeat 5 times on each side.

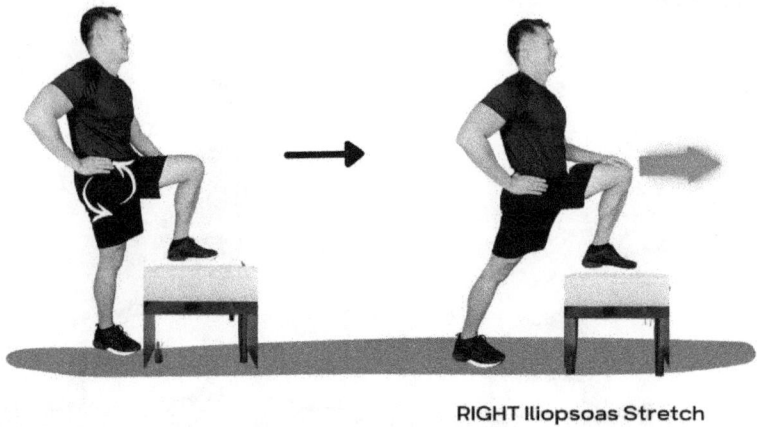

RIGHT Iliopsoas Stretch

Figure 11. Iliopsoas Stretch

1. While keeping your pelvis posteriorly tilted (see Step #2 of Iliopsoas Unlock), push your left knee forward as far as you can, stretching the tight iliopsoas muscle in front of your right hip.

2. Maintain the position and hold the stretch for 30 seconds.

3. Return to the original position.

4. Repeat 5 times on each side.

Hamstrings

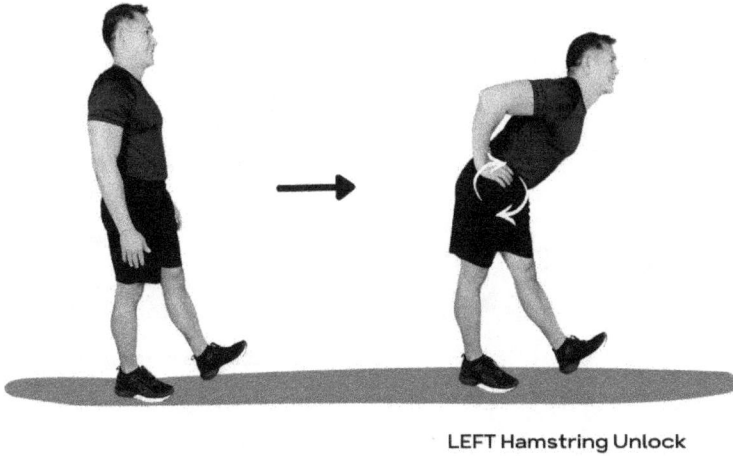

LEFT Hamstring Unlock

Figure 12. Hamstrings Unlock

1. Stand with one foot in front of the other.

2. Position the front foot with the heel on the floor and the forefoot and toes raised up.

3. Lean slightly forward and tilt your pelvis forward until you feel the stretch in your hamstring muscles.

4. Hold the stretch for 30 seconds.

5. Return to the original position.

6. Repeat 5 times on each side.

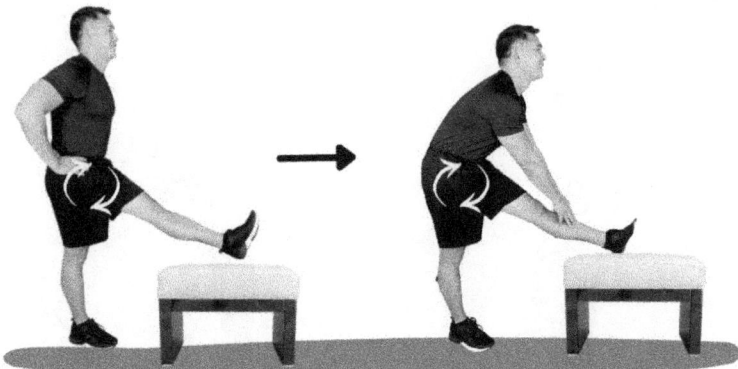

LEFT Hamstring Stretch

Figure 13. Hamstrings Stretch

1. While standing, place one foot on a chair with your knee extended.

2. Tilt your pelvis forward.

3. Lean forward until you feel the stretch on your hamstring muscles.

4. Maintain the position and hold the stretch for 30 seconds.

5. Repeat 5 times on each side.

Piriformis

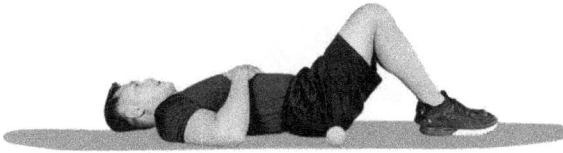

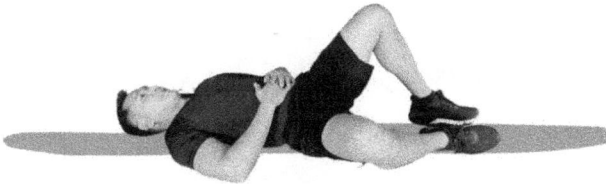

RIGHT Piriformis Unlock

Figure 14. Piriformis Unlock

1. Lie on your back.

2. Bend both knees up and put your feet flat on the ground.

3. Place a tennis ball in the middle of one butt cheek underneath your hip.

4. Draw one knee as far out as you can until you feel the stretch on your piriformis muscle.

5. Repeat 5 times on each side.

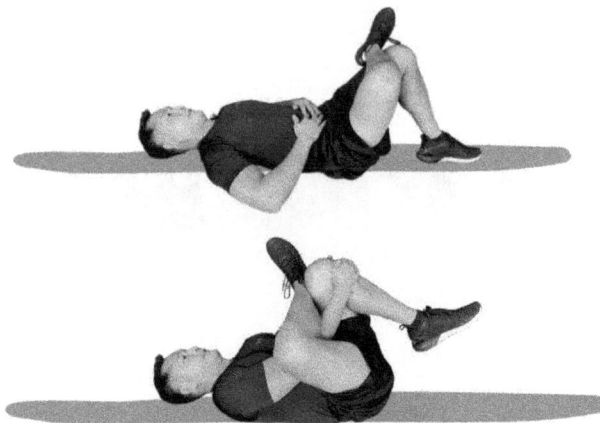

RIGHT Piriformis Stretch

Figure 15. Piriformis Stretch

1. Lie on your back.

2. Bend both knees up and put your feet flat on the ground.

3. Cross one leg up by placing the same leg on top of the other thigh.

4. Draw your knee up to your chest until you feel a stretch on your piriformis muscle.

5. Maintain the position and hold the stretch for 30 seconds.

6. Repeat 5 times on each side.

Social Component

Create an environment where you can maintain a consistent schedule and comply with the physical and cognitive activities of your back program.

1. Prior to starting your day/week, identify the best **days and *time*** for you to perform the physical and cognitive activities of your back program. If you don't allocate time for it, your busy schedule will take over your back program.

2. Identify a **place** where you can perform the cognitive and physical components of your back program. Ideally, the place you identify is where you can perform your back program with minimal distractions so you can focus on yourself and your needs, not the needs of the people surrounding you.

3. Identify a **person/group of people** who can give you "cues to action" and hold you accountable to your expressed schedule and goal.

KEY CHAPTER TAKEAWAYS

- You don't need to find a specific angle in your spine to achieve a pain-free, neutral spine position. As long as you are in the neighborhood, you are good!

- Determine your back's direction preference or bias to minimize the aggravation of your pain symptoms in the early stages of your recovery.

- Remember there are two reasons why your muscles may "lock up": *protective muscle tension* or *adaptive muscle tightness*. Use different techniques to remedy each one.

Chapter 11

Achieve Muscle Control and Spinal Stability
(STABILIZE Phase)

"You cannot always control what goes on outside.
But you can always control what goes on inside."

- WAYNE DYER

As you have learned in Chapter 6, the lumbar region of your spine is supported by a series of muscles that act as stabilizers. These muscles work together with the spinal or vertebral column, pelvis, and other structures to provide support for your back.

Unfortunately, fear that movement or physical activity may cause or aggravate your back pain will often limit or compromise your use of these muscles.[1] Additionally, prolonged bed rest or limited activity results in decreased or delayed activation and weakening of those muscles.[2-3]

There is evidence that your lumbar and abdominal muscles (multifidus and tranversus abdominis) contribute to lumbo-pelvic stability, segmental stiffness, and support of the spine when stability is challenged.[4] Therefore, achieving control and coordination of these muscles is critical to achieving fully sufficient spinal stability.

When these muscles contract, they create a stable base for all of your movements and physical function. If these muscles are weak or not coordinated, then it can lead to inadequate support and stability to your lumbar spine causing recurring low back pain or other injuries.

Learning how to activate these muscles properly through targeted physical activity is the secret to achieving the best support and stability for your low back.

Here's an example of the STABILIZE program using the framework you learned in the *Back Pain Unlocked System*™:

Cognitive Component

A key component in your journey to recovery is to think and truly believe that you're not broken or unfixable despite feeling a lot of pain. If you continue to think that you will never get better, the cognitive tools I am sharing with you cannot help.

These tools are designed to unlock the power of your mind, thereby reversing physical symptoms. If you don't believe that it's possible for all this to work, then it won't actually work at all.

Remember, pain neuroscience has taught us that our pain experience is informed and affected by our thoughts, beliefs, emotions, behavior, and attitude. The pain you are experiencing right now is your brain's opinion as informed by your subconscious thoughts and feelings.

Prior to performing the physical activities I outlined in this chapter, use a powerful cognitive tool psychologists call "self-talk".

Self-talk is your internal dialogue. It's influenced by your subconscious mind, and it reveals your thoughts, ideas, beliefs, and questions. If you've had low back pain for a while, your subconscious thoughts and beliefs about the physical activity will likely be skewed toward a negative bias. Your brain has been over-protective of you and does not want you to move. Doing the self-talk exercise I outlined below will help reframe your inner dialogue.

Instructions:

Using your own words, create a therapeutic self-talk. Make sure your self-talk feels natural and state it boldly and with authority. Finally, write it down on a piece of paper so you can read it repeatedly while performing the physical activities.

1. Determine who the message is intended for. Some find that talking to their pain helps, while others prefer to address their message to their body or mind.

2. Do not doubt what you know or have learned so far from your study of pain neuroscience. Tell your pain, body, or mind that you know what's going on, and you will not tolerate it this time.

   Example: *"Brain, I know that you are trying to protect me, but I am okay to do this physical activity. This will help me and not hurt me."*

3. Reassure your brain that you will address the issue. When you're feeling overwhelmed by emotion or find yourself in pain, tell your body that your back is inherently strong and is capable of handling physical activity.

   Example: *"Brain, I don't need pain to distract me right now. My back is strong and capable of performing this physical activity."*

4. Create a mental picture of the pain stopping. Close your eyes and visualize how you would like the pain to be gone. Imagine how it would feel if you were pain-free.

   Example: *Imagine a picture of the High Striker Tower and you're lowering the lever away from the alarm bells.*

If you really believe that this cognitive tool can help you, this activity can be a game-changer for you.

Physical Activity

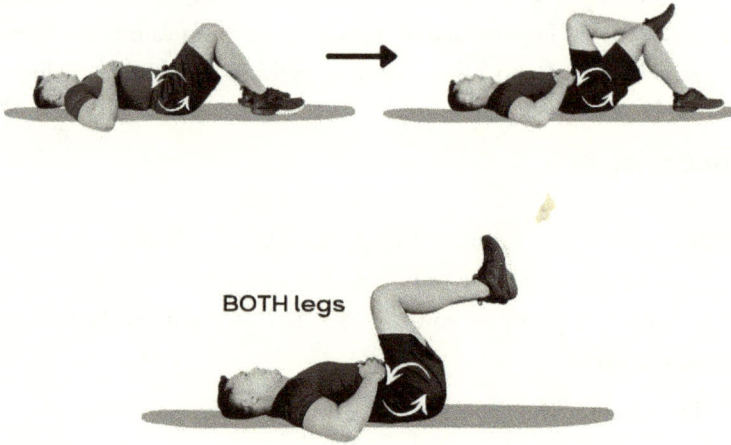

Figure 1. Tabletop Isometric Hold

1. Lie on your back with bent knees and the soles of your feet on the floor. In this position, the natural curve of your lumbar spine will lift the lower back slightly off the floor.

2. Exhale and slowly tilt your pelvis toward your head by engaging your abdominal muscles to pull your belly button back to your spine. As you do this, you'll feel your lower back pressing into the floor.

3. Once you've engaged your abs and tilted your pelvis, you will lift one foot up off the ground, bringing your knee directly on top of your hips.

4. Keeping your abdominal muscles engaged and your pelvis tilted toward your head, lift the other foot up off the ground, bringing your knee directly on top of your hips.

5. Keeping your abdominal muscles engaged and your low back flat on the floor, maintain the position for 5-10 seconds.

6. Slowly return to the original position.

7. Repeat 10 times.

Once you achieve mastery of this activity, progress to the next activity.

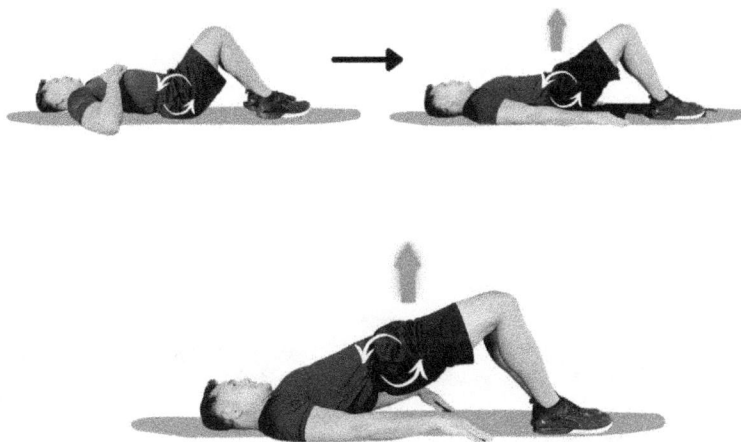

Figure 2. Segmental Bridge

1. Lie on your back with bent knees and the soles of your feet on the floor. In this position, the natural curve of your lumbar spine will lift the lower back slightly off the floor.

2. Exhale and slowly tilt your pelvis toward your head by engaging your abdominal muscles to pull your belly button back to your spine. As you do this, you'll feel your lower back pressing into the floor.

3. Starting from the bottom of your spine to your mid-back, and finally to your upper back, slowly "peel" your spine up from the floor until your hips are parallel to your knees.

4. Hold the position for 5-10 seconds.

5. Return to the original position.

6. Repeat 10 times.

Once you achieve mastery of this activity, progress to the next activity.

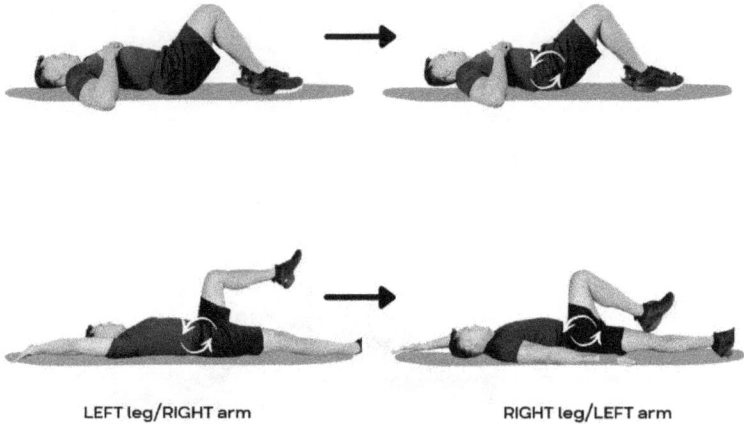

LEFT leg/RIGHT arm   RIGHT leg/LEFT arm

Figure 3. Dead Bug

1. Lie on your back with bent knees and the soles of your feet on the floor. In this position, the natural curve of your lumbar spine will lift the lower back slightly off the floor.

2. Exhale and slowly tilt your pelvis toward your head by engaging your abdominal muscles to pull your belly button back to your spine. As you do this, you'll feel your lower back pressing into the floor.

3. Once you've engaged your abs and tilted your pelvis, you will lift both feet up off the ground, bringing your knees directly on top of your hips.

4. Keeping your abdominal muscles engaged and your pelvis tilted toward your head, extend one knee while keeping the other knee on top of your hip.

5. Keeping your abdominal muscles engaged and your pelvis tilted toward your head, extend the other knee while keeping the first knee on top of your hip.

6. Make sure you keep your abdominal muscles engaged and your low back flat on the ground while alternately extending and flexing your knees.

7. Repeat 5 times on each side.

Once you achieve mastery of this activity, progress to the next activity.

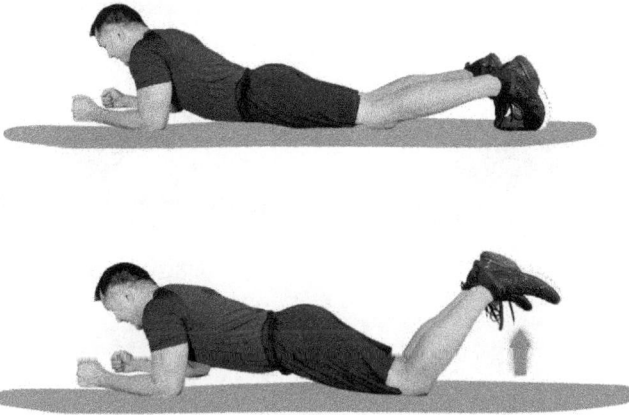

Figure 4. Plank on Knees and Elbows

1. Lie face down on the ground with your legs together and your arms at your sides.

2. Position your hands beneath your shoulders.

3. Tighten your core and elevate your upper body off the ground, stabilizing yourself with your forearms.

4. While keeping your knees down on the ground, raise your shin and feet off the ground.

5. Do not allow your hips to drop down. Hold the tension in your core for 30 seconds - 1 minute.

6. Slowly release back to the starting position.

7. Repeat 10 times.

Once you achieve mastery of this activity, progress to the next activity.

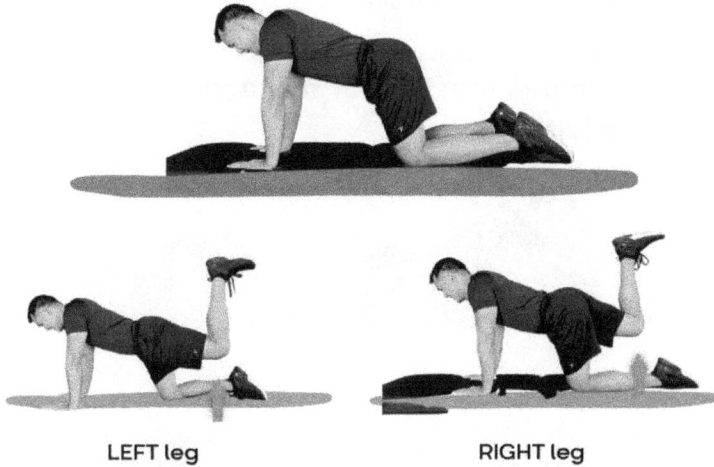

LEFT leg   RIGHT leg

Figure 5. Donkey Kick

1. Position yourself on all fours on a mat.

2. Position your hands underneath your shoulders and place your knees under your hips.

3. Keep your right knee bent at 90 degrees and extend your right hip until you lift the knee to the level of the hip.

4. Lower the knee without touching the floor and repeat the lift.

5. Once you've completed the reps on the right leg, switch legs.

6. Repeat 10 times on each side.

Once you achieve mastery of this activity, progress to the next activity.

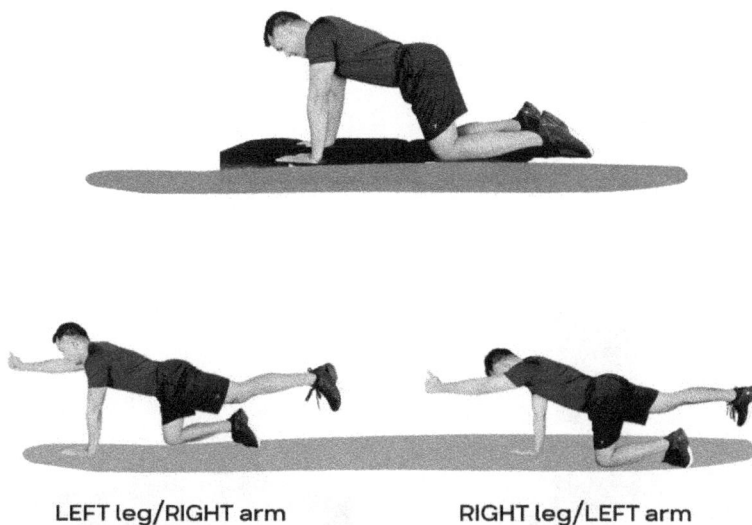

LEFT leg/RIGHT arm   RIGHT leg/LEFT arm

Figure 6. Bird Dog

1. Position yourself on all fours on a mat.

2. Position your hands underneath your shoulders and place your knees under your hips.

3. Brace your abdominal muscles.

4. Practice lifting one hand and the opposite knee just an inch or two off the floor while balancing on the other hand and knee and keeping your weight centered.

5. When you feel steady and ready to move on to a full range of motion, point the arm out straight in front and extend the opposite leg behind you. You should form one straight line from your hand to your foot, keeping your hips squared to the ground. If your low back begins to sag, raise your leg only as high as you can while keeping your back straight.

6. Hold for 5-10 seconds, then return your hands and knees.

7. Keep the abs engaged throughout the entire exercise, and work to minimize any extra motion in your hips during the weight shift.

8. Repeat 10 times on each side.

Once you achieve mastery of this activity, progress to the next activity.

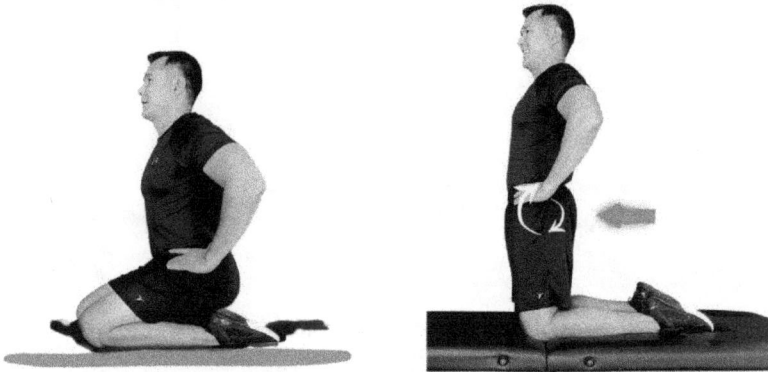

Figure 7. Tall Kneeling Hip Extension

1. Kneel on a mat or a pillow with your buttocks resting on your heels.

2. Transition into a tall kneeling position by squeezing your buttocks as tight as you can to extend your hips.

3. Simultaneously tilt your pelvis posteriorly as you squeeze your buttocks to extend your hips.

4. Return to the original position.

5. Repeat 15 times.

Once you achieve mastery of this activity, progress to the next activity.

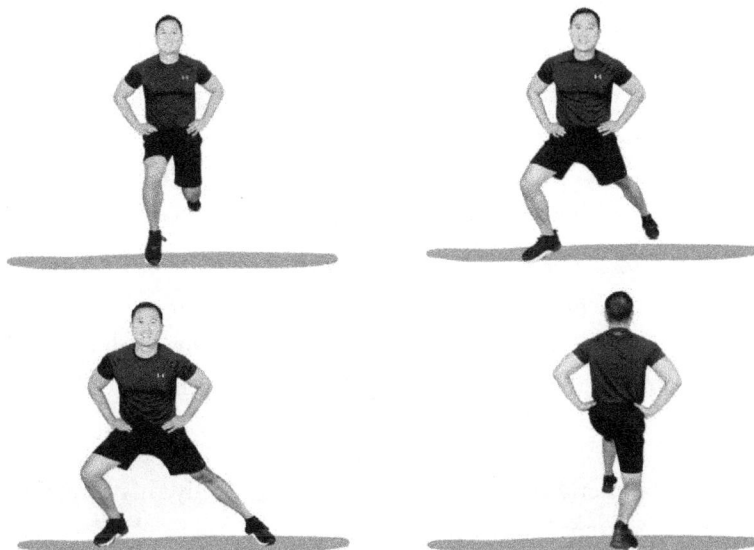

Figure 8. Multi-directional Lunge

1. Stand with your feet shoulder-width apart and fix your eyes, hips and toes all straight ahead.

2. *Forward lunge* - step forward with your right leg, placing your heel on the ground first. Then sink your hips until both knees bend at 90 degrees. Keep your abs and lower back braced, keep your upper body straight, and resist the urge to look down at any point.

3. Return to the original position.

4. *45-degree lunge* - Step out with your right leg again, this time at a 45-degree angle. Then sink your hips until both knees bend at 90 degrees. Keep your abs and lower back braced, keep your upper body straight, and resist the urge to look down at any point.

5. Return to the original position.

6. *Side lunge* - Step your right leg outwards at a 180-degree angle. You are not bending the left knee this time, just the right knee. Your left leg takes the strain in your groin when side lunging.

7. Return to the original position.

8. *Backwards 45-degree lunge* - Step backwards with the right leg at a 45-degree angle and drop your back knee towards the floor (without touching it). Note: Due to the natural way your foot will move here, your toes will come into contact with the floor before your heel, which is normal and safe.

9. *Backward lunge* - Step straight backwards with your right leg and touch the floor with your toes first. Lower your right knee towards the floor but do not touch it. This position is almost a direct reverse of the forward lunge. Bend both knees at 90 degrees.

10. Return to the original position.

11. Restart activity from the forward lunge, only this time with the left leg stepping out first.

12. Repeat 5 times on each side.

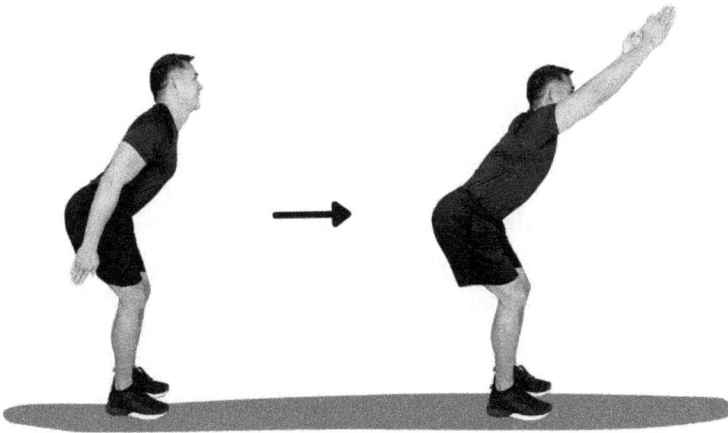

Figure 9. Hip Hinge with Back Extension

1. Stand with your feet shoulder-width apart.

2. Bend your knees slightly and keep your weight on your heels.

3. Lean forward by bending your hips while keeping your spine straight.

4. Lift your chest and push your buttocks backward.

5. Keep your head up, looking straight ahead.

6. Reach back with your arms and your shoulders pulling down toward your buttocks.

7. Hold this position for 10 seconds.

8. Keeping your position in step **#3**, lift your arms in front of you as high as you can.

9. Hold this position for 10 seconds.

10. Lower your arms back to your side and return to the original position.

11. Repeat 10 times.

Social Component

Write down the list of exercises I outlined above and give a copy to your accountability partner/s so they can provide you with reminders and cues to action on the days and times you committed to doing your back program.

See how we baked-in the cognitive and social components of your back program to your physical activity? That is why a comprehensive back program is more powerful and effective in the long-term than any one method or technique you may have tried before.

If you decide you want to add more variations and progressions to your physical activities, add different brain trainings to the cognitive component, and receive accountability prompts and coaching to fully implement the *Back Pain Unlocked System*™, you can book a call to chat with my team by going to:

BPUsystem.com/call

KEY CHAPTER TAKEAWAYS

- Fear of movement brought about by chronic low back pain will result in limited use or disuse of muscles essential to supporting and stabilizing your spine.

- Learning how to activate these muscles properly through a targeted physical activity is the secret to achieving the best support and stability to your low back.

- When you achieve muscle control and spinal stability, you create a stable base for all of your movements and physical function. When you don't, it can lead to inadequate support and stability to your lumbar spine causing recurring low back pain or other injuries.

Chapter 12

Achieve Long-Term Success
(MAINTAIN Phase)

*"Long-term success is a direct result of
what you achieve every day."*

RICK PITINO

As I mentioned in Chapter 4, any back program done an hour or two a day, no matter how efficient, is not sufficient to reverse the other twenty-two to twenty-three hours of faulty posture and movement patterns.

That is why the final phase of the *Back Pain Unlocked System*™ is the MAINTAIN phase. In this phase, I will teach you proper body mechanics and back care techniques to use throughout the day to optimize your long-term success.

Now that you know how to position your spine in its neutral, pain-free position (ALIGN) and use your back and abdominal muscles to brace your spine (STABILIZE), we'll build on what you've learned and apply it to your activities of daily living (MAINTAIN).

This is where everything you've learned so far comes together not just as a depository of information but as a skill set to be applied every day - this is the "do what you know" phase.

Here's the MAINTAIN phase following the framework you've learned from the *Back Pain Unlocked System*™:

Cognitive Component

Pain that lasts for more than three months is a sign of neuroplastic pain. Your brain becomes hypersensitive in this case and sends pain signals because it is on high alert trying to protect you. This is also called *chronic hyperalgesic state*.

Your brain remembers pain from past injuries and continues to trigger pain sensations even though the original injury has already healed.

When you live with chronic low back pain, it is hard not to think about it, and it's perfectly natural to worry that your pain might get worse if you go back to doing your usual activities of daily living.

That being said, we know from several studies that persistent negative thoughts and feelings about your experience of pain will only make your pain worse.[1]

In 1995, a team from Dalhousie University, a public research university in Nova Scotia, Canada, developed and validated a 13-item questionnaire that will help you assess your thoughts and feelings about pain.[2]

Read the statements below and decide for yourself whether these statements feel true for you. The only right answer is your honest answer so take your time to reflect on each statement.

When I am in pain...

- I worry all the time about whether the pain will end
- I feel I can't go on

- It's terrible and I think it's never going to get any better

- It's awful and I feel that it overwhelms me

- I feel I can't stand it anymore

- I become afraid that the pain will get worse

- I keep thinking of other painful events

- I anxiously want the pain to go away

- I can't seem to keep it out of my mind

- I keep thinking about how much it hurts

- I keep thinking about how badly I want the pain to stop

- There's nothing I can do to reduce the intensity of the pain

- I wonder whether something serious may happen

If you find that many of these statements sound similar to your own thoughts, don't worry. That just means your brain is using these thought patterns to form an opinion about pain.

By using psychosocial and behavioral tools that target cognitive processes, you can reprogram your nervous system and reduce the hypersensitivity of your alarm system.

Try this simple but effective cognitive exercise:

Replace out any wording that evoke negative mental images and emotions. Replace them with words that call upon positive thoughts and feelings.

For example, instead of saying *"My back hurts so bad."* or *"My back pain is flaring up."*, you could say *"I don't feel as comfortable right now."*

Even though you might not be comfortable, saying the word *"comfortable"* can make your brain's protective mechanism feel at ease, lowering down the volume of your alarm system.

Whenever possible, try to eliminate the use of the word "pain" to describe what you're feeling. Instead of describing how "painful" your back is, simply describe the sensation as a *"less comfortable"* feeling.

Saying the word "*comfortable*" to yourself can help make your brain's protective mechanism feel at ease. Anything that is not going to set off your alarm system and cause a panic in the brain is much better than the word "pain".

If your brain is processing these signals as "*sensation*" or something "*less comfortable*", instead of "pain", you will create a different experience for your brain and your body.

Apply this cognitive tool each time you perform the usual physical activities you did prior to the initial onset of your back pain.

Physical Component

Hip Hinge

One of the most important movement patterns you should learn and use in your activities of daily living is your ability to perform a hip hinge correctly.

A hip hinge movement pattern actively engages your posterior chain of muscles (your glutes and hamstrings) while keeping your spine in its optimum, neutral, and pain-free position.

Knowing how to correctly perform this maneuver will build the foundation for doing most of the physically challenging and demanding tasks your low back is subjected to on a daily basis, i.e., getting up from a low chair, picking up light objects from the floor, or lifting heavy objects from the floor.

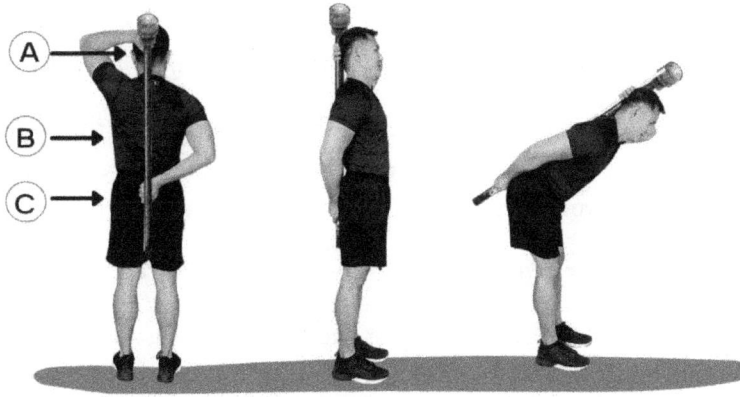

Figure 1. Hip Hinge

1. Stand with your feet shoulder-width apart.

2. Hold a dowel (or a broomstick, a golf club, or a cane) vertically behind your back with one hand on the top end and the other end by the bottom end.

3. The dowel should be in contact with the back of your head (A), center of your back (B), and bottom of your back (C) throughout the movement.

4. Start to learn forward by bending your hips and knees, bringing your shoulders and trunk forward.

5. Ensure the dowel always has a 3-point contact with your body.

6. Then, slowly bring the hips back to the starting position, ensuring the dowel always has a 3-point contact with your body.

7. Repeat 10-15 times.

Practicing this physical activity repeatedly will result in a sharp muscle memory you can utilize to confidently perform any activity throughout the day.

Pelvic Clock

How many times have you heard the command, *"Sit up straight!"*?

From the dining room admonitions you heard as a child to the computer screen reminders you have at your office, these reminders are ubiquitous - always ringing in your ears.

But why is it so hard to sit with your back straight *all the time*?

Because the muscles of your back, just like any of the muscles in your body that are subjected to a constant state of contraction, fatigue over time.

"Sit up straight all the time" is a nice reminder. It's just not a realistic expectation.

Just ask any office worker whose job requires them to sit in front of a computer for 6 or more hours in a day. Nobody can sit up straight *all* the time.

So, what will you do instead?

If getting up from your chair every 30-45 minutes is not feasible or practical, perform a pelvic clock instead.

Performing a pelvic clock every time you notice your low back getting tired from prolonged sitting is a great way to reintroduce movement to your spine and increase circulation around the periphery of your vertebral disc, decreasing the stress and strain to your low back.

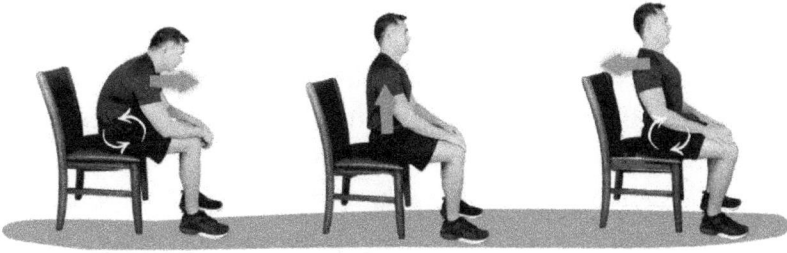

Figure 2. Pelvic Clock in Sitting

1. Sit in a comfortable position with your feet flat on the floor and your buttocks near the front of the seat.

2. Gently roll your shoulders forward. Feel the weight move backward on your "sit" bones and you tilt your pelvis backward toward the back of the chair.

3. Now straighten up slowly and pause at the mid-point (the neighborhood of your pain-free, neutral spine position!).

4. Now roll your shoulders back and extend your back and you tilt your pelvis forward toward the front of the chair.

5. Repeat 10 times every 30-45 minutes of prolonged sitting.

Sit to Stand

The ability to stand up from a chair without aggravating your back pain makes a huge difference in your activities of daily living. Essential functional activities, including getting up from a low toilet, out of bed, and out of a chair can be a distressing event if you are experiencing back pain. It doesn't have to be with this movement pattern I outline for you below.

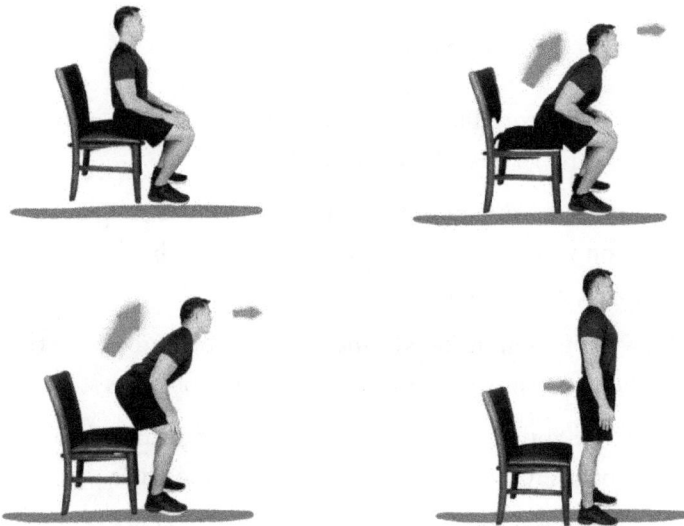

Figure 3. Sit to Stand

1. Scoot your hips forward to the edge of the chair.

2. Bring your *toes* underneath your knees.

3. Lean your body forward, *using the hip hinge technique*, while keeping your chest out and your gaze forward. (*Note:* looking down will round your upper back and counter the direction of your hip hinge.)

4. Extend your hips while pushing down on your feet to get into a standing position.

5. *Optional:* Use arms to push off the chair or off your knees.

Picking Up Light Objects from the Floor

This technique is also called "golfer's pick". This technique builds on the hip hinge technique (Figure #1) in that you are bending your hip joint while keeping your spine straight, decreasing the strain on your lumbar spine.

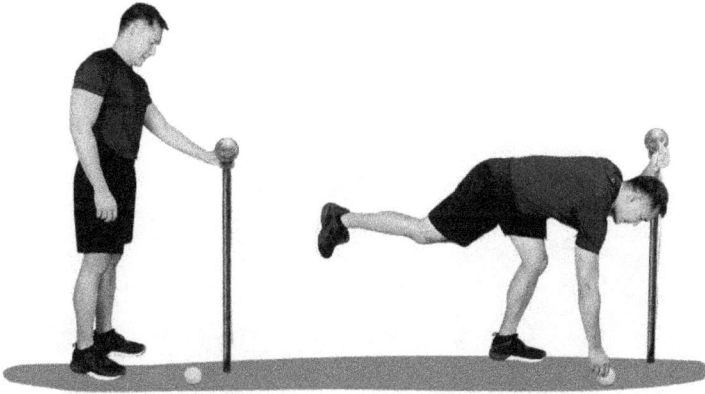

Figure 4. Picking Up Light Objects from the Floor

1. For this technique, the knees only slightly bend.

2. One leg is allowed to come off the floor behind the lifter and acts as a counterbalance.

3. The opposite hip bends and the body becomes almost parallel to the floor, except for the leg bearing your weight.

4. One arm reaches down to pick up the object while the other is often holding on to a stationary object for support, i.e., counter-top, chair, or a golf club or cane.

5. Although the chest does point down toward the floor, lifting the back leg allows the spine to stay straight and the counterbalance offsets the strain on the back.

Lifting Heavy Objects from The Floor

How many times have you heard people hurting their back after lifting a heavy object from the floor? Follow the movement pattern I outline below to avoid compressing your spinal discs or straining your lower back when you are lifting heavy objects.

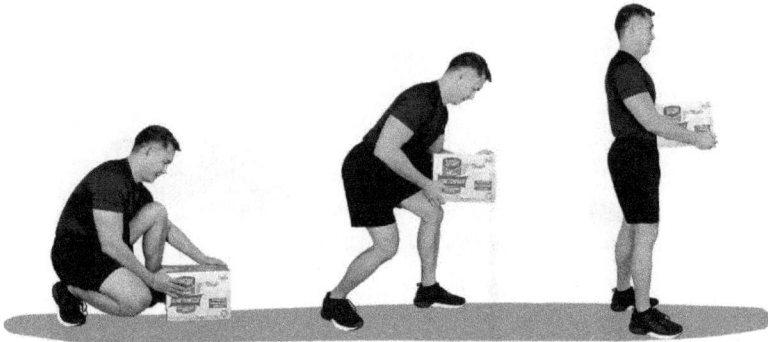

Figure 5. Lifting Up Heavy Objects from the Floor

1. Keep a wide base of support. Your feet should be shoulder-width apart, with one foot slightly ahead of the other (karate stance).

2. Squat down, bending at the hips and knees only. If needed, put one knee to the floor and your other knee in front of you, bent at a right angle (half kneeling).

3. Look straight ahead, and keep your back straight, your chest out, and your shoulders back. This helps keep your upper back straight while having a slight arch in your lower back.

4. Slowly lift by straightening your hips and knees (*not your back*). Keep your back straight, and *don't twist as you lift.*

5. Hold the load as close to your body as possible.

6. Use your feet to change direction or to turn; *do not twist your back.*

7. Set down your load carefully, squatting with the knees and hips only.

Do not attempt to lift by bending forward. Bend your hips and knees to squat down to your load, keep it close to your body, and straighten your legs to lift. Avoid turning or twisting your body while lifting or holding a heavy object.

Getting Up from the Bed

After several hours of sleep where your body is relatively less mobile, joint stiffness and muscle tightness may have set in that makes getting up and out of bed difficult.

In addition, the body mechanics of getting out of bed require transitional movements that often combine bending and twisting forces on your low back. Use the movement pattern I outline below to counter the effects of early morning low back stiffness and discomfort.

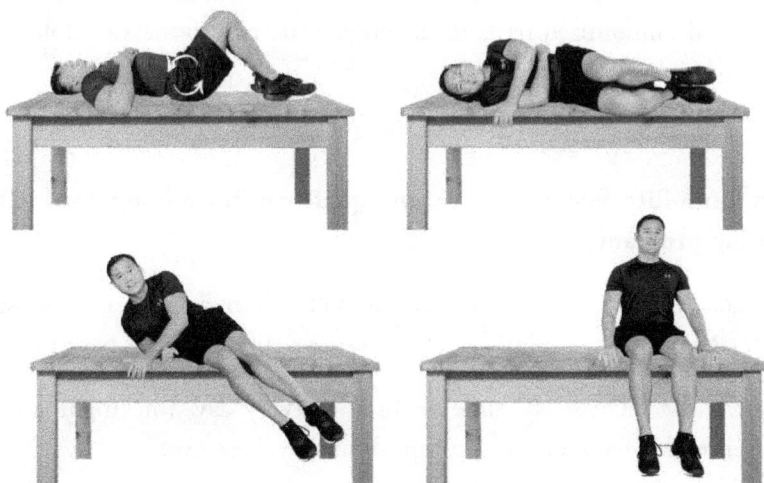

Figure 6. Getting Up from a Bed

1. The first step before transitioning from lying to sitting up in bed is to gently draw in your abdomen by pulling your belly button towards the bed. Maintain the abdominal drawing in maneuver while sliding one heel up at a time to bend both knees.

2. Keep your shoulders and hips in line with each other while turning onto your side.

3. This technique, referred to as *log rolling*, helps to reduce twisting and bending stress on the spine.

4. Once you are on your side, bend your knees so that your feet and lower legs are almost over the edge of the bed.

5. Now push into the bed with your top hand and bottom elbow while simultaneously allowing your feet to drop to the floor.

Walking

Finally, I would be remiss if I didn't advocate for the value of a walking program, both as a treatment and maintenance program for chronic low back pain.

In 2017, a team of researchers conducted a systematic review and meta-analysis of randomized trials to investigate the effectiveness of walking in chronic low back pain patients.

Their conclusion?

Pain, disability, fear-avoidance, and quality of life all improved with a walking program.

Set a goal of either time or distance you will walk in a day. Start with walking for 10 minutes, aiming for a heart rate of 100-110 beats per minute.

Progressively increase the time or distance every day. You might surprise yourself with what you can accomplish in a week or two.

And as you walk toward a life of freedom and function, let this old Chinese proverb encourage you, "A journey of a thousand miles begins with a single step."

Take your first step, my friend.

Conclusion

START YOUR

BACK PAIN UNLOCKED SYSTEM™

What To Do Next?

We've now reached the conclusion of this book and you now have the knowledge to treat your chronic low back pain at home. You now know more about your back than the hundred people who sit or stand next to you.

To recap what we've covered:

1. In the first chapter, we took a deep look at the research and evidence-based information on each of the current treatment options available to you today.

    We looked at the use of opioid pain medications and the risks of increasing drug tolerance, dependence, and/or addiction in using pain pills as the primary treatment of choice for chronic low back pain.

    We looked at the use of corticosteroid injections, its lack of long-term effect, and the resulting risk of osteoporosis with each succeeding shot taken.

We also studied the option of back surgery, the recommended indications for surgery, and the risk of failed back surgery syndrome (FBSS).

2. In the next few chapters, we looked into why a comprehensive back program like the *Back Pain Unlocked System*™ offers you the best chance to achieve a long-term solution to your chronic low back pain.

    We also looked at the hurdles and challenges many people encounter in implementing a comprehensive back program.

3. In Part 2, we studied the inherent anatomical and structural strength of your back, giving you confidence that your back is capable of the myriad movements and physical activities you will subject it to.

    We also looked at the common diagnoses seen in MRIs, X-Rays, and scans of the back, and their lack of correlation to pain and function.

    Finally, we studied the neuroscience of pain and the efficacy of using the biopsychosocial model in treating chronic low back pain.

    By the end, we had explored the different components (the three legs supporting a comprehensive back program) critical to helping you achieve the long-term solution of having a pain-free functional back.

4. Then we designed a comprehensive, logical, and well-coordinated program to include the different components critical to your success.

    You should now have a strong understanding of what you need to do to get started in setting up your own comprehensive back program.

5. Finally, in Part 3, we walked the map of the entire system.

You now have a 20,000-foot view of the system and you also know how to implement it from the ground up. We spent time looking at each component, implementing the necessary activity for each one.

The next step for you is simple:

Start.

Decide if you want help or if you want to do it alone but start.

If you do decide you want help, reach out to our team here:

BPUsystem.com/call

You deserve to live your life to the fullest.

Don't let chronic low back pain hold you back.

Your friend,

Dr. Lex Gonzales, PT, DPT

GLOSSARY

acute back pain - pain of less than one month duration caused by a specific disease or injury and resolves on its own or which has no long-term harmful effect on a person's health.

catastrophizing - to imagine the worst possible outcome of an action or event; to think about a situation or event as having a potentially catastrophic outcome. Catastrophizers are described as individuals who have a tendency to magnify or exaggerate the threat value or seriousness of the pain sensations.

cerebrospinal fluid (CSF) - a clear watery fluid that circulates around the brain and spinal cord and serves as a cushion or shock absorber for the central nervous system.

corticosteroid - resembles cortisol, a hormone naturally produced by the body's adrenal glands. They are mainly used to reduce inflammation and suppress the immune system.

chronic back pain - pain that continues for 3 months or longer, even after the initial injury or underlying cause of acute low back pain has been treated.

epidural - the space on or around the spinal cord.

hyperalgesia - abnormally heightened sensitivity to pain.

laminectomy - a surgical operation to remove the back of one or more vertebrae, usually to give access to the spinal cord or to relieve pressure on nerves.

meta-analysis - a statistical procedure for combining numerical data from multiple separate studies.

neurologic symptoms - results from injury or changes to the functioning of the brain, spine or nerves. The term 'neurologic' comes from neurology – the branch of medicine that deals with problems affecting the nervous system.

neuroscience - The study of the brain and nervous system, including molecular neuroscience, cellular neuroscience, cognitive neuroscience, psychophysics, computational modeling and diseases of the nervous system.

opioids - sometimes referred to as narcotics; a class of drugs naturally found in the opium poppy plant and that work in the brain to produce a variety of effects. Opioids can be prescription medications often referred to as painkillers, or they can be so-called street drugs, such as heroin.

osteoporosis - a medical condition in which the bones become brittle and fragile from loss of tissue, typically because of hormonal changes, or deficiency of calcium or vitamin D.

spinal fusion - a surgical operation to permanently connect two or more vertebrae in your spine, eliminating motion between them.

sprain - a stretching or tearing of ligaments — the tough bands of fibrous tissue that connect two bones together in your joints.

systematic review - a high-level overview of primary research on a particular research question that systematically identifies, selects, evaluates, and synthesizes all high-quality research evidence relevant to that question in order to answer it. In other words, it provides an exhaustive summary of scholarly literature related to a particular research topic or question.

Bibliography

Chapter 1

1. McCance-Katz, E. F., Sullivan, L., & Nallani, S. (2010). Drug interactions of clinical importance among the opioids, methadone and buprenorphine, and other frequently prescribed medications: A review. *American Journal of Addiction, 19*(1), 4–16. doi: 10.1111/j.1521-0391.2009.00005.x

2. AnGee Baldini, MD, Michael Von Koff, ScD, and Elizabeth H.B. Lin, MD, MPH. A review of potential adverse effects of long-term opioid therapy: A Practioner's Guide. Prim Care Companion CNS Disord. 2012; 14(3): PCC.11m01326. Published online 2012 Jun 14. Doi:10.4088/PCC.11m01326

3. Centers for Disease and Control and Prevention. 2018 Annual Surveillance Report of Drug-related Risks and Outcomes – United States. Surveillance Special Report 2. CDC, U.S. Department of Health and Human Services. Published August 31, 2018.

4. Rachel N. Lipari, Ph.D., Matthew Williams, Ph.D., and Struther L. Van Horn, M.A. Why do adults misuse prescription drugs? The CBHSQ Report, July 27, 2017

5. Opioid Overdose Crises, National Institute on Drug Abuse (NIDA) https://www.drugabuse.gov/drugs-abuse/opioids/opioid-overdose-crisis. Accessed June 2, 2019

6. Dowell D, Haegerich TM, Chou R. CDC Guideline for Prescrib-

ing Opioids for Chronic Pain – United States, 2016. MMWR Recomm Rep 2016;65(No. RR-1):1-49. DOI:http//dx.doi.org/10.15585/mmwr.rr6501e1

7. Fraser, Lisa-Ann, and Jonathan D Adachi. "Glucocorticoid-induced osteoporosis: treatment update and review." *Therapeutic advances in musculoskeletal disease* vol. 1,2 (2009): 71-85. doi:10.1177/1759720X09343729

8. Mandel S, Schilling J, Peterson E, Rao DS, Sanders W. A retrospective analysis of vertebral body fractures following epidural steroid injections. J Bone Joint Surg Am. 2013; 95: 961-4

9. https://www.fda.gov/drugs/drug-safety-and-availability/fda-drug-safety-communication-fda-requires-label-changes-warn-rare-serious-neurologic-problems-after Accessed March14, 2019

10. Chou R, Hashimoto R, Friedly J, et al. Pain Management Injection Therapies for Low Back Pain [Internet]. Rockville (MD): Agency for Healthcare Research and Quality (US); 2015.Available from: https://www.ncbi.nlm.nih.gov/books/NBK285206/

11. https://www.espn.com/nba/story/_/id/15148955/on-top-nba-world-steve-kerr-found-struggling-just-stand. Accessed June 20,2019

12. Kelvin WT. Electrical Units of Measurements. In: Kelvin WT. Popular Lectures and Addresses. London, England: Macmillan; 1899:73

13. Agency for Healthcare Research and Quality (AHRQ), Center for Delivery, Organization, and Markets, Healthcare Cost and Utilization Project (HCUP), Nationwide Inpatient Sample (NIS), 2001—2011

14. Thomson S. Failed back surgery syndrome – definition, epidemiology and demographics. Br J Pain. 2013;7(1):56–59

15. Harvey AM. Classification of chronic pain – descriptions of chronic pain syndromes and definitions of pain terms. Clin J Pain. 1995;11(2):163.7

16. Ragab, Ashraf et al. Management of Back Pain in Patients with Previous Back Surgery. *The American Journal of Medicine*, Volume 121, Issue 4, 72-278

17. https://www.washintonpost.com/news/early-lead/2017/04/24/how-agonizing-persistent-back-problems-are-thereatening-steve-kerrs-coaching-career. Accessed June 20, 2019

18. Jakobson Ramin, Cathryn. *Crooked: Outwitting the Back Pain Industry and Getting on the Road to Recovery.* Harper; 1 edition (May 9, 2017)

19. Hayden JA, van Tulder MW, Tomlinson G. Systematic review: strategies for using exercise therapy to improve outcome in chronic low back pain. *Ann Intern Med.* 2005 May 3;142(9):776-785

20. Koes BW, van Tulder MW, Lin CW, Macedo LG, McAuley J, Maher C. An updated review of clinical guidelines for the management of non-specific low back pain in primary care. *Eur Spine J.* 2010 Dec; 19(12):2075-2094. Epub 2010 Jul 3.

21. Bekkering, G.E., Hendriks, H.J., Koes, BW; Oostendorp, RA; Ostelo, RW, Thomassen, JM; van Tulder, MW. Dutch physiotherapy guidelines for low back pain. *Physiotherapy* 2003, 89, 82-96.

22. National Health Services (NHS). Back pain. Available online: http://www.nhs.uk/conditions/back-pain/Pages/Introduction.aspx (Accessed June 17, 2019)

23. Danneels, LA; Vanderstraeten, GG; Cambier, DC; Witvrouw, EE; de Cuyper, HJ. CT imaging of trunk muscles in chronic low back pain patients and healthy control subjects. *Eur Spine J.* 2000, 9, 266-272.

24. Youdas, JW. Lumbar lordosis and pelvic inclination in adults with chronic low back pain. *Phys. Ther.* 2000, 80, 261-275.

25. Kim, H; Chung, S; Kim, S; Shin, H; Lee, J; Kim, S. Influences of trunk muscles on lumbar lordosis and sacral angle. *Eur. Spine J.* 2006, 15,409-414.

26. Li, Y; McClure, PW; Pratt, N. The effect of hamstring muscles

stretching on standing posture and on lumbar and hip motions during forward bending. *Phys. Ther.* 1996, 76, 836-845.

27. Engel GL. The need for a new medical model: a challenge for biomedicine. *Science.* 1977; 196:129–136.

28. Engel GL. The clinical application of the biopsychosocial model. *Am J Psychiatry.* 1980;137:535–544.

Chapter 2

1. Low Back Pain: Clinical Practice Guidelines Linked to International Classification of Functioning, Disability, and Health from the Orthopedic Section of the American Physical Therapy Association. https://www.jospt.org/doi/pdf/10.2519/jospt.2012.42.4.A1 Accessed January 27, 2019

2. Mansour AR, Farmer MA, Baliki MN, Apkarian AV. Chronic pain: the role of learning and brain plasticity. Restor Neurol Neurosci. 2014;32(1):129-139. doi:10.3233/RNN-139003

3. Lunde LH, Nordhus IH, Pallesen S. The effectiveness of cognitive and behavioural treatment of chronic pain in the elderly: a quantitative review. J Clin Psychol Med Settings. 2009 Sep;16(3):254-62. doi: 10.1007/s10880-009-9162-y. Epub 2009 May 8. PMID: 19424781.

Chapter 3

1. Gatchel RJ, Peng YB, Peters ML, Fuchs PN, Turk DC. The biopsychosocial approach to chronic pain: scientific advances and future directions. Psychol Bull. 2007;133(4):581-624.

2. Straub RO. Health Psychology: A BioPsychosocial Approach. New York, NY: Worth Publishers; 2014.

Chapter 4

1. Deyo RA, Mirza SK, Martin BI. Back pain prevalence and visit rates: estimates from U.S. national surveys, 2002. *Spine.* Nov 1 2006; 31(23):2724-2727.

2. Maier-Riehle B, Harter M. The effects of back schools – a meta-analysis. *Int J Rehabil Res.* Sep 2001; 24(3): 199-206.

3. Chaves JE, Brown JM. Spontaneous cognitive strategies for the control of clinical pain and stress. J Behav Med. 1987;10(3):263-276.

4. Rosenstiel AK, Keefe FJ. The use of coping strategies in low back pain patients: relationship to patient characteristics and current adjustment. Pain. 1983;17(1):33-44.

5. Spanos NP, Radtke-Bodorik HL, Ferguson JD, Jones B. The effects of hypnotic susceptibility, suggestions for analgesia, and the utilization of cognitive strategies on the reduction of pain. J Abnorm Psychol. 1979;88(3):282-292.

6. Meichenbaum DH. Cognitive-Behavior Modification. New York, NY: Plenum Press; 1977.

7. Wertli MM, Eugster R, Held U, Steurer J, Kofmehl R, Weiser S. Catastrophizing—a prognostic factor for outcome in patients with low back pain: a systematic review. Spine J. 2014;14(11):2639-2657.

Chapter 5

1. George SI. What is the Effectiveness of a Biopsychosocial Approach to Individual Physiotherapy Care for Chronic Low Back Pain?. The Internet Journal of Allied Health Sciences and Practice. 2008 Jan 01;6(1), Article 4.

Chapter 6

1. Kimble C. Health in America. *Wilson Q.* 1980 Spring:60-101.

Chapter 7

1. Elliot JM, Flynn TW, Al-Najjar A, Press J, Nguyen B, Noteboom JT. The pearls and pitfalls of magnetic resonance imaging for the spine. *The Journal of Orthopedic and Sports Physical Therapy.* Nov 2011; 41(11):848-860.

2. Videman T, Battie MC, Gibbons LE, Maravilla K, Manninen H, Kaprio J. Associations between back pain history and lumbar MRI findings. *Spine.* Mar 15, 2003;28(6):582-588

3. Kjaer P, Lebouf-Yde C, Korsholm L, Sorensen JS, Bendix T. Magentic resonance imaging and low back pain in adults: a diagnostic imaging study of 40-year-old men and women. *Spine.* May 15 2005;30(10):1173-1180.

4. Alyas F, Turner M, Connell D. MRI findings in the lumbar spines of asymptomatic, adolescent, elite tennis players. *Br J Sports Med.* Nov 2007;41(11):836-841; discussion 841.

5. David Hanscom MD *Back in Control: A Surgeon's Roadmap Out of Chronic Pain* Vertus Press; 2nd ed. edition (November 18, 2016)

Chapter 8

1. Moseley L. Combined physiotherapy and education is efficacious for chronic low back pain. *Aust J Physiother.* 2002;48(4):297-302

2. Louw A, Diener I, Butler DS, Puentedura EJ. The effect of neuroscience education on pain, disability, anxiety, and stress in chronic musculoskeletal pain. *Archives of physical medicine and rehabilitation.* Dec 2011; 92(12):2041-2056.

3. Gatchel RJ, Peng YB, Peters ML, Fuchs PN, Turk DC. The biopsychosocial approach to chronic pain: scientific advances and future directions. *Psychol Bull.* 2007 Jul;133(4):581-624. doi: 10.1037/0033-2909.133.4.581. PMID: 17592957.

4. Nielson WR, Weir R. Biopsychosocial approaches to the treatment

of chronic pain. *Clin J Pain*. 2001 Dec;17(4 Suppl):S114-27. doi: 10.1097/00002508-200112001-00020. PMID: 11783824.

5. Carter R. *The Human Brain Book*. First ed. New York: Dorling Kindersley Limited; 2009

6. Puentedura EJ, Louw A. A neuroscience approach to managing athletes with low back pain. *Phys Ther Sport*. Aug 2012; 13(3):123-133

7. Louw A, *Why Do I Hurt?* A Neuroscience Approach to Pain. Minneapolis:OPTP; 2013

8. Louw A, Butler DS, Diener I, Puentedura EJ. Development of a preoperative neuroscience educational program for patients with lumbar radiculopathy. *American Journal of Physical Medicine & Rehabilitation / Association of Academic Physiatrists*. May 2013; 92(5):446-452.

9. Louw A. *Your Nerves Are Having Back Surgery*. Minneapolis: OPTP; 2012

10. Vlaeyen JW, Linto SJ. Fear-avoidance and its consequences in chronic musculoskeletal pain: a state of the art. Pain. Apr 2000;85(3):317-332

11. Abdallah CG, Geha P. Chronic Pain and Chronic Stress: Two Sides of the Same Coin? *Chronic Stress*. February 2017. doi:10.1177/2470547017704763

12. Jennings EM, Okine BN, Roche M, Finn DP. Stress-induced hyperalgesia. *Prog Neurobiol*. 2014 Oct;121:1-18. doi: 10.1016/j. pneurobio.2014.06.003. Epub 2014 Jul 8. PMID: 25010858.

Chapter 9

1. Fares MY, Fares J, Salhab HA, Khachfe HH, Bdeir A, Fares Y. Low Back Pain Among Weightlifting Adolescents and Young Adults. *Cureus*. 2020;12(7):e9127. Published 2020 Jul 11. doi:10.7759/ cureus.9127

2. Siewe J, Rudat J, Röllinghoff M, Schlegel UJ, Eysel P, Michael JWP. Injuries and overuse syndromes in powerlifting. *Int J Sports Med.* 2011;32:703–711.

3. Lederman E. The Myth of Core Stability. *CPDO Online Journal.* June 2007:1-17.

Chapter 10

1. Lloyd DM, Helbig T, Findlay G, Roberts N, Nurmikko T. Brain Areas Involved in Anticipation of Clinically Relevant Pain in Low Back Pain Populations With High Levels of Pain Behavior. J Pain. 2016 May;17(5):577-87. doi: 10.1016/j.jpain.2016.01.470. Epub 2016 Feb 1. PMID: 26844417.

2. Linton SJ. Chronic back pain: integrating psychological and physical therapy--an overview. Behav Med. 1994 Fall;20(3):101-4. doi: 10.1080/08964289.1994.9934623. PMID: 7865928.

Chapter 11

1. Karayannis NV, Smeets RJEM, van den Hoorn W, Hodges PW (2013) Fear of Movement Is Related to Trunk Stiffness in Low Back Pain. PLoS ONE 8(6): e67779. https://doi.org/10.1371/journal.pone.0067779

2. Hodges P and Richardson C. Inefficient muscular stabilization of the lumbar spine associated with low back pain. A motor control evaluation of transversus abdominis. *Spine* 1996 21: 2640-2650.

3. Ferreira P, Ferreira M, Maher C, et al. Changes in recruitment of transversus abdominis correlate with disability in people with chronic low back pain. *Br J Sports Med* 2010;44 1166-1172

4. Hides J, Stanton W, Mendis M, et al. The relationship of transversus abdominis and lumbar multifidus clinical muscle tests in patients with chronic low back pain. *Man Ther* 2011; 16: 573-577

Chapter 12

1. Lumley MA, Cohen JL, Borszcz GS, et al. Pain and emotion: a biopsychosocial review of recent research. *J Clin Psychol.* 2011;67(9):942-968. doi:10.1002/jclp.20816

2. Sullivan M. J.; Bishop S. R.; Pivik J. (1995). "The Pain Catastrophizing Scale: Development And Validation". *Psychological Assessment.* 7 (4): 524–532. CiteSeerX 10.1.1.323.7545. doi:10.1037/1040-3590.7.4.524

About the Author

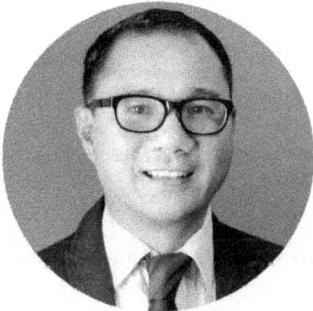

Dr. Lex Gonzales, PT, DPT is the Amazon bestselling author of THE BOOK OF BALANCE: Rehab Secrets to Improve Your Balance and Decrease Your Risk of Falling and winner of the 12th National Indie Excellence Awards, Nonfiction Category.

He has been a physical/physiotherapist for over twenty-four years with a special interest in the field of geriatric rehabilitation. He received his degree of Doctor of Physical Therapy from the University of South Florida and his certification as a Vestibular Rehabilitation Therapist from the American Institute of Balance.

He is certified by Stanford University as an instructor of Empowered Relief™, a transformative pain treatment that rapidly equips patients with pain management skills.

While working as Director of Rehabilitation for a national health and rehabilitation company, Dr. Gonzales received the CORe certification in Business Analytics, Economics for Managers, and Financial Accounting from HBX, Harvard Business School.

He lives with his wife and two daughters on the northeast coast of Florida, USA.

Visit him at drlexgonzales.com

FINALLY, A SENSIBLE AND EFFECTIVE SYSTEM TO HELP YOU ACHIEVE A PAIN-FREE, FUNCTIONAL BACK!

Back Pain Unlocked is loaded with research and evidence-based information and proven strategies to treat your persistent, recurring, or chronic low back pain. The Back Pain Unlocked System™ is a comprehensive and well-coordinated system that follows the biopsychosocial model of treatment to address the different components of your chronic pain experience.

In this content-rich book, you will learn the answers to:

- What is your back's directional preference or bias?
- What is the meaning of your X-ray, MRI, or CT scan result?
- What is the percentage of "Failed Back Surgery Syndrome?"
- What is the effect of steroid injections to your vertebral bones?
- How to locate your spine's optimum, pain-free position?
- What is your body's living pain alarm system, and how to turn down its hypersensitivity to pain?

What You Are About to Discover from This Book is the Same System That Allowed My Patients to Live Their Best Selves - Achieving the Quality of Life They Richly Deserved!

Dr. Lex Gonzales, PT, DPT is a public speaker and award-winning author who has been a physical/physiotherapist for over twenty-four years with a special interest in the field of geriatric rehabilitation. He received his degree of Doctor of Physical Therapy from the University of South Florida and his certification as a Vestibular Rehabilitation Therapist from the American Institute of Balance. He is certified by Stanford University as an instructor of Empowered Relief™, a transformative pain treatment that rapidly equips patients with pain management skills.

Visit him at drlexgonzales.com

www.ingramcontent.com/pod-product-compliance
Lightning Source LLC
Chambersburg PA
CBHW020002290326
41935CB00007B/275